The Female Profile of Autism

from the same authors

The Autism Spectrum, Sexuality and the Law
What Every Parent and Professional Needs to Know
Tony Attwood, Isabelle Hénault and Nick Dubin
ISBN 978 1 84905 919 0
eISBN 9780 8 5700 679 0

Asperger's Syndrome and Sexuality
From Adolescence through Adulthood
Isabelle Hénault
Foreword by Tony Attwood
ISBN 978 1 84310 189 5
eISBN 978 1 84642 235 5

of related interest

Women and Girls on the Autism Spectrum, Second Edition
Understanding Life Experiences from Early Childhood to Old Age
Sarah Hendrickx with Jess Hendrickx
Foreword by Dr Judith Gould
ISBN 978 1 80501 069 2
eISBN 978 1 80501 070 8
Audiobook ISBN 978 1 39980 729 6

Working with Girls and Young Women with
an Autism Spectrum Condition
A Practical Guide for Clinicians
Fiona Fisher Bullivant
ISBN 978 1 78592 420 0
eISBN 978 1 78450 784 8

THE FEMALE PROFILE OF AUTISM

A GUIDE TO CLINICAL ASSESSMENT

ISABELLE HÉNAULT
and **ANNYCK MARTIN**

in collaboration with
Tony Attwood, **Valentina Pasin** and **Bruno Wicker**

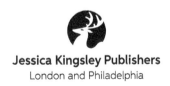

Jessica Kingsley Publishers
London and Philadelphia

First published in French in Canada in 2021 by Chenelière Education
First published in English in Great Britain in 2025 by Jessica Kingsley Publishers
An imprint of John Murray Press

2

Copyright © 2021 TC Média Livres Inc. Translation

Translated by Rebecca du Plessis

The right of Isabelle Hénault, Annyck Martin, Tony Attwood, Valentina Pasin
and Bruno Wicker to be identified as the Authors of the Work has been asserted
by them in accordance with the Copyright, Designs and Patents Act 1988.

It's Raining on My Dreams! © Isabelle Queyroi-Mallet 2018
Foreword © Tony Attwood 2025

Front cover image source: Apolline Silary. The cover image is for
illustrative purposes only, and any person featuring is a model.

A CIP catalogue record for this title is available from the
British Library and the Library of Congress

ISBN 978 1 83997 828 9
eISBN 978 1 83997 829 6

Printed and bound in Great Britain by Clays Ltd

Jessica Kingsley Publishers' policy is to use papers that are natural,
renewable and recyclable products and made from wood grown in
sustainable forests. The logging and manufacturing processes are expected
to conform to the environmental regulations of the country of origin.

Jessica Kingsley Publishers
Carmelite House
50 Victoria Embankment
London EC4Y 0DZ

www.jkp.com

John Murray Press
Part of Hodder & Stoughton Limited
An Hachette UK Company

The authorised representative in the EEA is Hachette Ireland,
8 Castlecourt Centre, Dublin 15, D15 XTP3, Ireland (email: info@hbgi.ie)

Contents

Part 2: Story of an Adult Diagnosis   77
ANNYCK MARTIN

Part 3: Guidelines for the Clinical Assessment and Diagnosis of Autism in Female Adolescents and Adults   131
TONY ATTWOOD, ISABELLE HÉNAULT, VALENTINA PASIN AND BRUNO WICKER

Appendices

Foreword

TONY ATTWOOD

Recently, clinicians have seen an increase in the number of women and girls seeking an autism diagnosis. The ratio was previously estimated to be four autistic boys and men to every autistic girl or woman. Currently, clinical and research experience is showing a ratio more like two to one. Requests for diagnostic assessment for girls and women come from various sources, notably parents and caregivers,[1] spouses and partners, schools and mental health services.

The clinical profile of autism in girls is often very subtle during the first years of primary school but becomes more apparent towards the end of primary and the start of secondary school. During this time, social skills and friendships increase in complexity and abstraction. An autistic girl will feel increasingly different to the other girls, and the adaptation strategies she adopts as a result of her autism and her psychological response to her feeling of isolation may contribute to the development of a variety of behavioural and mental health problems, leading to an assessment for autism.

Three psychological adaptation strategies are seen in autism. An autistic child will resort to the first strategy when they feel overwhelmed, unsettled or uncertain of social situations, particularly while playing with or speaking to their peers. An autistic child, and especially an autistic girl, is all too aware of the risks of making a social faux pas, being ridiculed or feeling stupid. As a coping mechanism, autistic girls might actively avoid all social interactions and take refuge in their

---

1   Where we refer to 'parents' throughout the book, we include caregivers and guardians.

imagination, which they can control and enjoy more easily. In these cases, they will be seen as introverted and extremely shy.

Nonetheless, some autistic children are more extroverted. They feel motivated to engage in social relationships, but given their difficulties in 'decoding' signals and social contexts that determine, regulate and moderate social interactions, their behaviour can be seen as intrusive, impulsive and annoying. The two adaptation strategies mentioned so far can be concerning to parents and teachers, who will initiate a process of diagnostic assessment looking to explain why a child would choose to isolate themselves socially or interact with others with no awareness of social conventions or signals that seem all too obvious to their peers.

A third adaptation strategy in autism, only recently recognized by clinicians and researchers, and initially identified in autistic girls and women, consists of being keen to build social relationships but first abstaining from these relationships while observing and closely analysing the social interactions of others. In this way, they will decipher social conventions and work out some 'scenarios' of play and conversation, and then use this information and adapt their behaviour for a given social setting. We now recognize that many autistic girls and some autistic boys will use this adaptation, which efficiently camouflages or masks social difficulties using imitation, and projects sociability and reciprocity. However, it proves hugely draining because this strategy works cognitively rather than intuitively, although it is very effective and will delay a diagnostic assessment.

To adopt this masking strategy, an autistic child must turn themselves into a mini psychologist or scientist in search of social rules, clues and responses, as illustrated in the following quote from an autistic woman: 'As a child, I was often copying other people (kids at school, storybook characters, TV characters, etc.) in the hopes that the copied behaviors would win me the approval of others. Only it didn't work, as my timing and deliverance was off. Plus there was the issue of too little or too much' (quoted in McKibbin 2015, p.39).

At home, the autistic child will likely observe and explore the thoughts, feelings and social conventions of family and peers, and become an avid reader of fiction that describes the social behaviour of children of the same age. At home, there may be play with dolls and figurines to recreate social experiences from school, which helps analyse and decode social behaviours. An autistic teenager might watch television series or films to help decode and learn about social scenarios for future use. The autistic teenager will progressively become an expert in imitation, wearing a social 'mask' that can hide autism. The young autistic adult who camouflages their autism gives the impression of being non-autistic, and their performance becomes genuinely Oscar-worthy. As one young autistic woman said: 'I did such a good job of pretending to be normal that nobody really believes I have Asperger's' (quoted in McKibbin 2015, p.40). But all this comes at a price. An autistic person who uses this third adaptation of observation, analysis and imitation can feel that to be accepted and avoid being rejected, they have to suppress their autistic characteristics, not be their authentic self, and create a new persona and identity.

The repression of autistic characteristics and true identity first emerges as a coping strategy at school. An autistic child can seem to their teachers to be a quiet and studious pupil, not easily distracted by social interactions, and keen to please their teachers. There can be a fear of negative judgements, as much from teachers as from their peers, and an autistic girl may try hard to maintain a positive and harmonious atmosphere in class and in the playground. By contrast, when she comes home, she can be a completely different person, becoming volatile, hypercritical and confrontational. Her parents long for her to be the same person at home as at school.

Clinicians recognize that some autistic girls develop artistic talents, notably in the visual arts, while some are talented singers, musicians or fiction writers. Some have an aptitude for languages and become multilingual. Some have an incredible gift for working with animals, or can become highly skilled in the caring professions, such as nursing, medicine or psychology.

In some cases, over the years, young autistic women can develop almost a 'sixth sense' that enables them to perceive and absorb the negative moods of others, especially anxiety, agitation or despair. It is possible that the social withdrawal associated with autism might not just be attributable to a lack of social skills or unpleasant sensory experiences, but is perhaps also a means of self-protection to avoid getting 'contaminated' by other people's negative mood patterns.

Another means of adaptation for autistic girls can take the form of a preference for playing with boys. One autistic woman explained that, when she was a child, 'a lot of the stereotyped activities associated with girls were stupid, boring, and inexplicable' (quoted in McKibbin

2015, p.129). She added: 'The girls' behaviour was more elaborate and mean-spirited than I could understand' (McKibbin 2015, p.131). From an autistic girl's point of view, it is easier to work out what you have to do when playing with boys because the games tend either to be active or construction-based, as when playing with LEGO®-style building blocks, rather than based around conversations and emotions in the course of which subtle facial expressions such as 'eye rolls' must be interpreted. Consequently, an autistic girl can become a 'tomboy' and actively invest her time in sports and boys' games. Nonetheless, it is also possible that she will avoid playing with boys just as much as girls, instead seeing her pets as trusted friends who are genuinely happy to see and be with her.

During adolescence, puberty entails physiological, cognitive and emotional changes, and friendships take on new dimensions. One of the characteristics of autism is an aversion to changes and transitions, in such a way that an autistic girl can struggle to adapt to the changes in her body as she becomes a woman, preferring to stay young or androgynous. She has difficulty understanding and adapting to the shifting expectations of her teenage peers, and she might have problems showing interest in the same things as others, particularly in the area of relationships.

Autistic girls can try to be accepted by other girls by becoming overtly feminine in their clothes and interests – for example, by developing a special interest in make-up and femininity, regular topics of conversation among their peers. However, if this strategy doesn't work during adolescence, the pendulum can swing back, and an autistic girl can become disdainful of femininity and gender roles, looking instead to associate with those who favour gender neutrality or who are sometimes more socially marginalized.

Adolescence is when feelings of identity or sense of self are explored on the journey to adulthood. Unfortunately, for autistic adolescents, their sense of self can often rest on a fragile identity, particularly if they have had to mask to become more popular by artificial means. Highly emotionally draining, masking can contribute to clinical depression as a result of autistic burnout. On the other hand, people who don't mask their autistic traits can build an identity based more on the criticism and rejection of their peers than on compliments and acceptance. This can lead to low self-esteem and a fragile sense of identity, which can also contribute to clinical depression.

There is a strong link between autism and anxiety. During adolescence, this anxiety can grow considerably and cause one or more serious mental health problems, notably conditions such as generalized anxiety disorder, obsessive-compulsive disorder, social anxiety disorder, phobias linked to specific sensory experiences or performance anxiety, and especially a fear of making mistakes. Episodes of situational mutism can occur due to extremely high levels of anxiety in certain social situations. Clinical diagnostic assessment for anxiety disorders or depression in teenagers should include a detailed developmental history in which the clinician takes into account all behaviours and skills associated with autism. There is also a link between autism and eating disorders, borderline personality disorder, gender dysphoria and substance abuse. Clinicians specializing in a range of diagnoses in teenagers and young adults should, therefore, envisage autism as a possibility and make every effort to identify it.

Requests for autism assessment by grown women have also increased. To arrive at the point of looking for a diagnosis, they might have received an autism diagnosis for their child and find they recognize traits and experiences from their childhood; they might have had problems in their relationships or at work; or they might have learned about autism in the media. A diagnosis can bring a massive sense of relief when they finally discover the reasons they have always felt different without ever knowing why. Autistic women, more than autistic men, often have a keen sense of the positive aspects of their autism – for example, their ability to see the world differently; their capacity to concentrate on detail, on repeating patterns, or errors; their artistic and creative streak; as well as their more extraordinary powers of empathy, social justice and compassion. They can also be determined to help other autistic women, perhaps even by speaking of their experiences in an autobiography.

Finally, the clinical assessment guide in Part 3 of this book combines in-depth experience of diagnoses and therapeutic support services based on the most recent studies on the female profile of autism. This guide contains information on the new diagnostic tools used for screening autism, the latest procedures for seeking a diagnosis, and therapeutic support for autistic people throughout their lives. Here, at last, is the guide clinicians need, and that autistic people would like to see them read and explore.

Acknowledgements

ISABELLE HÉNAULT

First, I would like to thank Professor Tony Attwood, my mentor and friend for 15 years now. Our meeting changed the course of my life. As a result of his generosity and hospitality in Brisbane, Australia, I was able to gain clinical experience and expand my knowledge, by means of total immersion. He knew how to transmit his passion for autism, and I will forever admire his outstanding abilities as a clinician.

Thanks to Annyck Martin for her generous contribution. As soon as the idea for this book came along, I immediately asked her to be my co-writer because her life course and her determination moved me. Her rich and sensitive inner life deserves to be brought to light through her narrative, by reading her thoughts, her story and her research. A gifted writer (among many other gifts!), she is a real treasure of a co-author.

Thanks to France D and Isabelle Queyroi-Mallet, who agreed to share their experiences. This is admirable, to my mind, because it demonstrates a level of trust, in addition to sending a message of hope to autistic women. Thank you so much, Isabelle, for your patience and for your truly monastic work editing the manuscript. Your eagle eye and your exceptional skills as a writer make you a unique colleague. Meeting you has been as enlightening on a personal front as it has been for me professionally. I thank you sincerely for all that you are.

Thanks to Valentina Pasin, my Italian friend and colleague. Our year together in the clinic in Montréal was emotional and full of experiences. Your sensitivity, your intelligence and your personality make you a wonderful psychologist. Your major contribution to the clinical assessment guide enriches both this book and the wider field of female autism.

A huge thank you to my partner who, with his patience, advice and support, enabled me to accomplish this project and many others... And thank you also to my sunshine, my son, who makes me laugh and appreciate life every day.

A special thank you to Apolline Silary for her artwork, which is on the front cover of this book. Our meeting was truly a gift, and it inspired me to write about the beauty and richness of autistic women.

Finally thank you to all the autistic women who inspire me every day. I have so much respect for you and your lives. I dedicate this book to you.

ANNYCK MARTIN

I would like to thank Francis, Anaïs and Nanou for being there and for their unconditional love and support. Isabelle, for our co-writing adventure and for our shared desire for awareness about autism in girls and internal presentations of autism. Caroline, for our discussions, her support and for her sense of humour. France D and Isabelle Queyroi-Mallet, for sharing their rich experiences. All autistic and neurodivergent people, for their strength and resilience. My friends and acquaintances, for inspiring me. The professionals who seek to learn, understand and improve their practice with autistic women and girls, to provide them with better support and contribute to changing their lives for the better.

Preface

ISABELLE HÉNAULT

ASD: autism spectrum disorder

ASC: autism spectrum condition

Having been a clinician for 18 years, I have met many autistic adults. Previously, it was a majority of boys and men I saw for consultation. Six years ago, my practice changed following the publication of clinical questionnaires and assessment grids from the psychologist community on female autism, and in response to a growing demand from women looking for an accurate diagnosis and tailored ongoing support. I quickly became interested in these women, who had been sidelined from autism spectrum disorder (ASD) and, above all, had been incorrectly diagnosed, frequently with personality disorders or bipolar disorder.

As a psychologist, I have been able to meet women from across the world to improve my understanding of the traits, the characteristics they have in common, that make up female autism. As in many Western countries, the profession of psychologist is recognized on several levels in Québec. Since 2012, depending on their training, qualifications and areas of expertise, psychologists are able to diagnose and provide psychotherapy services. This eases the burden on public health services, offers a more dedicated service and gives us the ability to work in multidisciplinary teams. The benefits of this are numerous, as much for autistic women as for clinicians.

With the help of renowned scholars and clinicians in the field (Tony Attwood, Valentina Pasin and Bruno Wicker), we have been able to devise a diagnostic tool as well as a comprehensive clinical guide to autism in women and girls. I am sharing my experience to increase recognition of this condition in women, in the hope of improving their access to appropriate support, which might lead to a better quality of life for these women.

This book responds to a real need in France, Québec and elsewhere, anywhere that autism spectrum disorder is still misunderstood and little supported.

Introduction

'And what if autism was considered alongside the female profile?' These were the words of Christopher Gillberg, a Swedish specialist in autism, at an international conference several years ago.

Long thought to be a majority male condition, level 1 autism, or Asperger's syndrome, is a condition that has been well documented since the publication of *Asperger's Syndrome: A Guide for Parents and Professionals* by Tony Attwood in 1998. Several questionnaires and diagnostic tools have been developed and then scientifically approved in different countries. For a long time, a ratio of four or five autistic boys or men to every one autistic girl or woman has been put forward in the scientific literature (Moore 2023). The predominantly male criteria provide an explanation as to why many women only identify partially with the characteristics and behaviours that are usually described.

In the last 10 years, several blogs and autobiographical books by autistic women have appeared. Clinically, women have started to question their specificities and similarities without having received an autism diagnosis. However, since 2011 researchers and clinicians specializing in autism have become interested in the female profile and have begun adapting grids and questionnaires (e.g. Attwood 2012; Kopp and Gillberg 2011). Today, the ratio has moved to three men to every woman (Loomes *et al.* 2017), and clinically we are now seeing a ratio of two men to one woman, or even one to one.

THE AIMS OF THIS BOOK

The main objective of this book is to demystify female autism. It is also aimed at giving credence to the experiences of women who suspect they have this condition, and to avoid the often-inaccurate diagnoses by professionals who misunderstand the particularities of the male and female profile. Additionally, in covering a variety of subjects and suggested interventions, it is hoped that this book might also enable girls and women to achieve a quality of life in line with their abilities and potential.

THE STRUCTURE OF THE BOOK

In Part 1 we define female autism and present its clinical criteria and the associated subjects it is important to tackle, especially sexuality, relationships, professional life and, finally, the route to diagnosis. Part 2, by Annyck Martin, will tell the story of a life with autism from the inside. Annyck's story illustrates her route to discovery of the condition in herself, and what happened next... Finally, Part 3 contains the clinical assessment guide for female autism. A detailed questionnaire provides an oversight of the characteristics unique to women and others who mask. It is based on the diagnostic questionnaires and clinical data gathered as a result of collaboration with Professor Tony Attwood, neuropsychologist Valentina Pasin and neuroscience researcher Bruno Wicker. This unique tool will guide both professionals and autistic adults, with its detailed description of the traits and characteristics of autism in women.

The three worksheets (from Chapters 4 and 6 in Part 1) and the Appendices in Part 3 can be photocopied or downloaded from https://digitalhub.jkp.com/redeem using the code BUVNZAM.

WHO THIS BOOK IS FOR

The book is written for a wide readership, particularly girls and women who think they recognize the autistic profile in themselves and might be autistic, autistic women themselves, as well as professionals working with autistic people or who are interested in the subject of autism in women and girls.

This includes:

- Mainstream and special educational needs teachers of any level

- Guidance counsellors

- School psychologists, educational psychologists and clinical psychologists

- Special education technicians

- Child psychiatrists and psychiatrists

- Social workers

- Doctors.

The clinical assessment guide in Part 3 is aimed more towards professionals, enabling them to give access to assessment, as well as to psychologists, doctors and psychiatrists who are able to make an official diagnosis.

The women's accounts in this book are full of emotion, and illustrate the difficult path to obtaining an official diagnosis – an outcome that would provide recognition and also give access to an identity. Here is a first account by a woman telling the story of her path.

FRANCE D'S STORY

Before. Wandering:

Like being inside a too-small diving suit, walking the tightrope of life.

Razor-sharp worry, quicksand of anxiety.

Avoidance, flight, run-for-your-life.

Guilt, the shame of being different to others.

Fascination with birds, would have liked to be one, probably to fly away more easily.

Allergic to celebrations, get-togethers, ceremonies, small talk, parties, even my own.

Relentless mental turmoil when faced with the array of uncontrollable possibilities.

Human relationships? Being surrounded by mousetraps with no means of escape.

Huge difficulty making connections. Constant feeling of rejection.

Hate small talk, empty and superficial conversations.

Intensity of feelings and emotions, but struggle to express them.

I feel the feelings of others as if they were my own; it's exhausting.

Concern for justice and equity to the point of obsession. Keen intolerance of injustice.

Incapable of saying anything but the truth.

Sensitive to the woes of the world, from the age of six.

Hyperaesthesia: especially sight, smells, sounds.

Still feel like a child, even now.

My appearance doesn't matter to me. I like to be comfortable.

Yes, I followed fashion for a while, and wore high heels even though I couldn't bear them.

Behind me:

Well, I don't remember much before the age of three.

As a young child, I liked anything that spinned. Said to be a difficult, capricious, stubborn child, painfully shy, mute outside the family home.

Would have liked to be a boy, from the age of six or seven... because there are too many injustices for girls. Why is it up to girls to do the washing up? Boys eat too, don't they?

At school, very split between my intense desire to learn and my unease at being in a class of 30 little girls. Often faked illness so as not to have to go. Playtime was torture, too much stimulation, shouting, movement. Even today, if I walk past a playground during break, I have a surge of anxiety. Group tasks were painful. I preferred by far to work alone. I never completed the Cégep [the Montréal school leavers' certificate]; it was intolerable for me to be in a group.

So books became my best friend.

In primary school I understood everything straightaway without needing to make any effort. Very different in secondary school.

Algebra and chemistry turned me off completely: whatever did numbers have to do with letters? It made no sense to me. Needless to say, I hated those subjects.

Since I was a child, I have been fascinated by the world, by its highest mountains. I dreamed of travelling, of an elsewhere where I could simply be happy.

During adolescence, I had no idea how to behave around boys. Which ended in an unplanned pregnancy at the age of 18. I was naive, and I didn't know what I wanted from life, let alone what I wanted from boys. At 18, I had the maturity of a 13- or 14-year-old.

Indifferent to my own life, which I found no more important than a breadcrumb. What was it for? Who was it for? I only wanted one thing: to be accepted, to be loved, despite the huge chasm separating me from others. I frequently wanted to be invisible, to disappear.

Female friendships? A mystery. I only ever had one friend, from 4 to 17 years old. I spent most of my time alone with my books, puzzles, drawings and stamp collection, especially in the summer when my only friend would go to her holiday house. Occasionally, I was invited along, to my delight/dismay... Yes, I'm with her, but I'm not at home. I loved being outside, in the woods, alone, my precious birdsong the only soundtrack. Childhood trauma: often, when I was boisterous/disobedient, I heard 'We'll send you to boarding school', which would literally make me freeze, as if electrocuted. I never understood parents' codes, 'We don't say that', 'We don't do that', 'What will people think?'

A sense of intuition, a sixth sense, I can inexplicably sense things as if I had sensors.

Incapable of sleeping in the same bed as anybody else.

Worse...not even in the same room either! The breathing, and the body movements.

Not having any filters, I can end up saying something too personal, which can shock people. I can't help it. Nothing is taboo to me.

I like everything to be organized, tidied away, even inside the dishwasher. It makes me feel secure. When things are in disarray I don't feel well mentally, which leads to anxiety.

Unpleasant feelings, such as having wet feet, can make me furious.

False diagnosis of bipolarity... Fluctuating between overstimulation and depression. Antidepressants, hospitalizations, occasional brushes with death. Five or six years ago...big turning point. I decided to stop my medication and stop seeing psychiatrists, and do my own research. After all, at the age of 60, who knows me better but myself?

With the help of a shrink I start an intense internal exploration, starting with my hypersensitivity. Having always been interested in psychology, I start reading about autism, that mysterious cavern... and...what if it was that? Despite everything, I'd had a seemingly 'normal' life, married with children. I got married twice, 28 years apart. Two ceremonies: good God, how I wished for those days to be over! As for work, I nearly always worked in the civil service: filing and more filing, how I loved that! I like when everything is tidy, ordered, in its right place, to the point of obsession.

I filed, I classified, all alone in my corner, peacefully. It was only the meetings and office meals that were unbearable for me. I never went for lunch with the other girls.

I can't abide obsequious people. I recently changed financial advisor. I can't bear to be called 'Madame' every 10 words!

I have lost friendships I relied upon, for speaking out of turn. Even though what I said made sense, and was logical and true.

I travelled a lot, just as I had dreamed of when I was seven or eight. At that age I knew all the capital cities of the world by heart. Strangely, I felt more at ease in countries where I didn't know the language than in Québec, where my inability to communicate was an obstacle. I didn't feel judged.

However, big cities frightened me, especially the underground rail, Montréal, Paris, St Petersburg, Delhi: too many people, noises, smells, the movement of crowds. I did manage to cope with it, though, so motivated was I to discover new countries. I always loved – and still love – world music.

My interests are medicine, psychology, travel, drawing, painting, since forever. I have had other interests too, very intensely for three or four years, before I move on to something else.

Nowadays, I am watching the film of my life with fresh eyes. Since my diagnosis in 2017, at the age of 64, I feel alive again...it's a revelation. I finally understand who I am. I have confidence in myself like never before. Quite simply, I am one of a rare breed of humans. I'm even proud of it. A blast of fresh air, or water in the desert...my horizons are finally opening up.

I feel like a freshly baked croissant, straight out of the oven.

And now?

So, relieved at my diagnosis, I want to have my moment in the sun, for the first time in my life. I tell people I am autistic; I don't have anything to lose apart from prejudices. Yes, that's what I am, take it or leave it! I want to educate people about this condition, which I don't consider to be an illness or disability.

And relationships? Yes, those who accept me and my quirks, my tendency to speak my mind, my haphazard thoughts, how intense I can be. As for the rest? They're out! Thanks to social networks

I have got to know other autistic women; we feel so at ease with each other. I also suspect that my partner is autistic. I delight in being alone, I take care of my needs. I set boundaries too, having been weak in the past. I always run away, it's true, but it has become very important to me to protect myself. To tame anxiety – I never say 'my' anxiety – I practise meditation. I am done with masking. I can finally begin to live the best years of my life knowing who I am!

Yes! So happy to be me!

PART 1

AUTISM: TO THE HEART OF THE FEMALE PROFILE

ISABELLE HÉNAULT

APA: American Psychiatric Association

ASC: Autism spectrum condition. A more positive term to describe autistic traits, rather than using the term 'disorder', which has a negative connotation

ASD: Autism spectrum disorder. ASD replaced the term pervasive developmental disorder (PDD) in the *Diagnostic and Statistical Manual of Mental Disorders, Fifth Edition* (DSM-5)

DSM-5-TR®: At the time of writing, the latest of the APA's *Diagnostic and Statistical Manual of Mental Disorders*, published in 2022

Gender dysphoria: A strong and permanent feeling of incongruity between gender assigned at birth and gender identity, causing psychological suffering, significant distress and compromised functioning in society

OCD: Obsessive-compulsive disorder

PDD: Pervasive developmental disorder

CHAPTER 1

The Autism Spectrum Definitions and Diagnostic Criteria

The *Diagnostic and Statistical Manual of Mental Disorders, Fifth Edition* (DSM-5) gives a full definition of autism spectrum disorder (APA 2013), and classes autism as a neurodevelopmental disorder.

The collective term autism spectrum condition (ASC) designates a group of neurodevelopmental conditions characterized by difficulties with social interactions, verbal and non-verbal communication, as well as repetitive behavioural patterns and areas of special interest. Typical behavioural manifestations are often present before three years old, but can also appear for the first time during the school years or later in life. Linked symptoms can vary considerably in nature and in intensity, even in the same person over time, and can be accompanied by other closely related diagnoses (or co-morbidities).

According to the DSM-5, the autism continuum consists of classic autism (Kanner's syndrome), considered to be level 3; level 2, which requires significant support and intervention; and level 1, which was previously considered to be 'high-functioning autism' or Asperger's syndrome.

AUTISM SPECTRUM OR ASPERGER'S SYNDROME?

Asperger's syndrome was renamed in the DSM-5 as ASD level 1, and is now designated as a form of autism with lower support needs. However, some clinicians and researchers in the field prefer to retain the label Asperger's, as given in the DSM-IV (APA 2000). On the one hand, the label enables the clear differentiation of classic autism, which is often accompanied by intellectual disabilities or the absence of speech, from high-functioning autism. On the other hand, among pervasive developmental disorders (PDD), Asperger's syndrome was only belatedly recognized in the nomenclature of *The ICD-10 Classification of Mental and Behavioural Disorders: Clinical Descriptions and Diagnostic Guidelines* (WHO 1993) and the DSM-IV.

Some existing members of the Asperger's (or Aspie)[1] community feel it offers a unifying definition for adults as well as providing a unique identity and an awareness of Aspie culture, avoiding confusing terms such as 'mild autism', 'classic autism' and 'high-functioning'. We also consider ASD to be a difference, not a deficiency. This framing guides my practice and the recommendations I make, which are adapted to the profile of skills and talents seen in autistic individuals. In this I am aligned with research and practice in the domain of neurodiversity.

A HISTORY OF ASPERGER'S SYNDROME

The Austrian psychiatrist Hans Asperger was the first to describe the syndrome in detail in 1944 (Asperger 1988). He used his observations of children in his clinic to describe different autistic conditions. His conclusions differed from those of Kanner (1943), who worked on classic autism. It is only in 1981, with the publication of Lorna Wing's article 'Asperger's Syndrome: A clinical account' in the journal *Psychological Medicine*, that the scientific community became aware of Asperger's syndrome. Then, in 1991, Uta Frith translated Asperger's original article into English. It's since the publication of this latter document that the scientific community has really focused its attention on this form of autism.

Since 2000, clinicians and autistic adults alike have become interested in the subject, and practical guides have started to be published. For example, in 1998, Professor Tony Attwood wrote *Asperger's*

---

1   The term 'Aspie' is one favoured by a majority of people in the Asperger's community, because a true Aspie culture has formed over the last few years.

Syndrome: A Guide for Parents and Professionals, a key reference in the field. Liane Holliday Willey, who has Asperger's, has written numerous fascinating autobiographical books, notably *Pretending to Be Normal: Living with Asperger's Syndrome (Autism Spectrum Disorder)* (1999), *Asperger Syndrome in the Family: Redefining Normal* (2001), and *Safety Skills for Asperger Women: How to Save a Perfectly Good Female Life* (2011). There has also been Rudy Simone's *Aspergirls: Empowering Females with Asperger Syndrome* (2010), and more recently, Julie Dachez, with *Invisible Differences: A Story of Asperger's, Adulting, and Living a Life in Full Color* (2020). In Québec, Marie Josée Cordeau has made a name for herself with a range of activities (a blog, a book, an information guide, a television series, etc.), and campaigns for recognition of the profile and for services adapted to the needs of women and girls.[2] These authors' reflections on Asperger's are pertinent and helpful for professionals, and for women seeking answers to why they are different.

For his part, Professor Attwood (2005b, 2008) considers that high-functioning autism (level 1 autism in the DSM-5) and Asperger's syndrome are found on the same continuum. He advocates for a search for commonalities between the two states, with a view to developing intervention programmes that are accessible to the autistic population as a whole. His thinking is along similar lines to that of Lorna Wing (1981), who asserts that certain so-called 'classic' autistic people progress towards Asperger's, especially if they have benefited from early intervention.

DIAGNOSTIC CRITERIA FOR AUTISM SPECTRUM DISORDER

Here is a synthesis of the diagnostic criteria for ASD:[3]

- Persistent difficulty with social communication and interactions

- Difficulty in social-emotional reciprocity

- Difficulty with non-verbal communicative behaviours used for social interaction

---

2   See https://mjcordeau.blogspot.com
3   There is a very useful article by the Indiana Resource Center for Autism, which cites the DSM-5's diagnostic criteria for autism: www.iidc.indiana.edu/irca/learn-about-autism/diagnostic-criteria-for-autism-spectrum-disorder.html

- Struggling with developing, maintaining and understanding relationships

- Restricted, repetitive patterns of behaviour, interests or activities

- Repetitive motor movements

- Insistence on sameness and/or inflexible adherence to routines or ritualized behaviour

- Highly fixated interests that are abnormal in intensity or focus

- Hyper- or hyposensitivity to sensory input.

In addition to the formal criteria, clinical observations will complete the diagnostic table:

- Social isolation: Shows little interest in interpersonal relationships.

- Communication: Fails to decode non-verbal language, and exchanges can more take the form of a monologue than a two-way conversation. There may be neologisms (words invented by the individual).

- Facial expressions, stereotypies: These take the form of tics, repetitive body movements, etc.

- Imagination and thought theory (or mind theory): Cognitively, the level of development of autistic people allows them to engage in symbolic play; however, they show deficiencies with regard to thought theory. According to Howlin, Baron-Cohen and Hadwin (1999), this theory is defined by an ability to attribute a certain mental state to oneself and to others. For example, just because I like drawing doesn't mean that everyone else likes drawing. I can enjoy an activity, but someone else might prefer another activity. For adolescents, I often explain that they can desire or feel attracted to someone, but it is not necessarily reciprocated. In terms of thoughts, I may find it easy to visualize numbers and do mental arithmetic, but it's not necessarily the same for everyone.

    This capacity for meta-representation usually develops around the age of four, but for autistic people, this development is delayed. Symbolic representations are idiosyncratic above all in the sense that they are specific and exclusive to the individual.

The other characteristics associated with ASD are linked to:

- Sensory responses (hypo- and hypersensitivity – one of the senses is frequently more developed than the others, and acts as a guide)

- Motor functions (impaired fine motor skills and coordination, in terms of body language, gait, movements, play, etc.)

- Impaired executive function (planning, organization, flexibility, emotional regulation)

- Emotions (they are hard to decode both in oneself and in others).

CHAPTER 2

Understanding the Characteristics of Autism

The autistic profile includes several characteristics, seen as much in men as in women. It is important to have a good understanding of the clinical characteristics associated with autism because they will clarify the necessary tools and required interventions. For example, if social conventions are badly understood or badly interpreted, this risks exacerbating social awkwardness.

SOCIAL SKILLS

It is important to mention here the research of Professor Tony Attwood and Carol Gray (2004). According to the studies that they reported on, almost 70 per cent of autistic young people experience bullying at school, and this increases symptoms linked to social anxiety. Some young adults start avoiding social contact through fear of ridicule and as a result of painful past experiences. Social withdrawal is often prioritized at the expense of joining groups or participating in social experiences.

It is important to teach social skills organically (in real-life situations) in order to increase the opportunity for encounters and conversations in a positive setting. In this way, feedback from friends, colleagues or family members will increase an individual's motivation to socialize. My clinical experience shows that many autistic people prefer to socialize in an organized context, particularly via the intermediary of a fun activity or a club, or in a context that lets them interact with others around an activity or a common interest. The feeling of pleasure and involvement then reduces social anxiety and fosters a positive experience.

Communication is made up of both verbal and non-verbal aspects: intonation, gestures, emotions, body language, etc. The verbal component constitutes the essence of the exchange. Autistic people can have difficulty decoding non-verbal communication, which explains misunderstandings and obstacles to reciprocal communication. Furthermore, verbal exchange may often be one-directional, because the discussion is often based on a special interest. The autistic person can passionately monopolize the conversation with a monologue or a detailed discussion about their field of interest.

The aim of the proposed interventions is to teach reciprocal communication. I often use the example of ping-pong or tennis, since the aim of these sports is for the ball to get to either end, in an exchange. So we need to teach the autistic person to ask questions, reflect, use non-verbal gestures (nodding in agreement, smiling, etc.) and give feedback to their interlocuter. Too often, and mistakenly, a lack of interest is detected by the interlocuter, because the autistic person rarely shows their interest by means of non-verbal language, verbal feedback or eye contact, which may be evasive or even non-existent.

TO FIND OUT MORE

The book by Don Gabor, *How to Start a Conversation and Make Friends* (2011) includes a plethora of practical, useful examples to help develop conversational skills, both verbal and non-verbal.

EMPATHY AND THEORY OF MIND

Theory of mind is the capacity to imagine thoughts, emotions and another person's intentions. A delay is observed in the development of these skills in autistic people. On the other hand, this does not mean that they don't have any empathy. While non-autistic people often express empathy by means of words and affectionate gestures, autistic people are more likely express empathy with their actions (helping someone to fix a computer, cooking a meal, finding solutions to a problem, etc.).

For autistic people, the difficulties linked to decoding and emotional regulation as well as theory of mind are, to some degree, responsible for the differing types of empathy. Totally absorbed in their special interest, they pay no attention to external stimuli.

The logical, practical way in which autistic people think can be equally problematic in an emotional context. News of an illness, the death of a loved one, loss of a job or any other event apt to provoke strong emotions in their partner may be translated into logical terms by the autistic person (e.g. 'Never mind', 'Ask your doctor', 'So it goes', 'It wasn't the job for you', 'You're making a big deal of it', 'So, what next?'). The partner or interlocuter will have the – incorrect – impression that the autistic person is insensitive to what they are going through, which risks creating conflict.

Empathy presents in three forms: cognitive empathy, emotional empathy and compassion. Cognitive empathy is the ability to 'know' what the other person is feeling – which doesn't imply kindness or any emotion towards the other. Emotional empathy is what most people are referring to when they talk of 'feeling what the other person is feeling'. Compassion, for its part, is the action that follows on from emotional experience (giving a kiss, making a gesture towards the other person, etc.).

Facial expressions and empathy are interlinked. Ekman (cited in Foreman 2003) defines empathy as a sophisticated ability to treat others as we would wish to be treated ourselves, based on early imitation. Imitation of facial expressions develops from an early age, but remains impaired in autistic people. Compassion towards animals is also found in certain autistic women. An unconditional attachment is described in these cases, as well as a sensitivity towards animals. This constitutes one of the characteristics of the 'sixth sense', which is defined as a hypersensitivity and feeling towards animals and certain people.

HYPERSENSITIVITY AND HYPOSENSITIVITY

Some autistic people may be hypo- or hypersensitive, depending on the sense (smell, hearing, touch, sight, taste, vestibular/balance, proprioception and interoception) (Bogdashina 2012; Côté 2016). A more developed sense may also act as a guide for the other senses.

Hypersensitivity

Hypersensitivity can be described as the extreme sensitivity of one or more of an individual's senses. In terms of sexuality, the five basic senses (hearing, smell, touch, taste and sight) are also very important. Auditory and tactile hypersensitivities are very common among autistic people, and may be associated with a neurological disorder (Bogdashina 2012). For example, background music might be perceived to be loud and invasive, even when the volume is on the lowest setting. Similarly, merely brushing against the skin can provoke the same level of pain as touching a sharp object. Brushing against the skin and contact with certain materials can cause a painful response. By contrast, pressure against the skin (in some cases, strong pressure) is often found to be calming (Aquilla 2003). Oversensitivity can hinder an intimate relationship developing, because a variety of stimulations can provoke discomfort and even be painful. An avoidance of all contact can increase a feeling of isolation and amplify depressive symptoms.

Hyposensitivity

Hyposensitivity is defined as a weak sensory response to stimuli, which feel inconsequential. In these cases, an overexposure to the stimuli is required in order to help the individual feel them in their entirety. For example, cold temperatures may not be felt very often; conversely, extreme heat doesn't inconvenience the person even though it may be very intense on a hot day. Many autistic people wear the same clothes all the year round, since they hardly feel the change in temperature. Aquilla (2003) explains these reactions as the result of a slow transfer of sensations from the nerve endings in the skin to the brain.

Temple Grandin, in her book *The Autistic Brain* (2014, with R. Panek), proposed an interesting hypothesis by which autistic hypersensitivity and hyposensitivity may have the same common root: hypersensitivity. It is sensory overload that causes hyposensitivity, as a sort of protection mechanism.

TO FIND OUT MORE

In their book *Asperger Syndrome and Sensory Issues*, Brenda Smith Myles and her colleagues (2000) reported on the incidence among people with Asperger's of sensitivities in emotions and in interpersonal relationships. They propose several different interpretations for sensory responses, and avenues for intervention adapted for each sense.

In her book *Favoriser l'attention par des stratégies sensorielles*, Sonya Côté (2016) offers a practical guide with exercises and tools that help rebalance sensory overload, bearing in mind the vestibular/balance system and proprioception. This is a very useful guide, since the exercises are the same for both children and adults.

CHAPTER 3

Understanding the Key Features of the Female Profile of Autism

I gained my first professional experience in Brisbane, Australia, in Professor Tony Attwood's clinic. Professor Attwood is a world authority on autism, and he has been working for more than 30 years in the field. Throughout his career he has met hundreds of children and adults. At diagnostic assessment sessions, we are seeing more and more women calling on the services of his clinic, hoping to get some clarity on their personality profile. At international conferences, too, numerous women have been asking him about a possible female profile, but with characteristics and subtleties as yet little documented in the scientific literature. Professor Attwood's works and reflections have led to the elaboration of a profile among autistic girls and women. Following on from this, an adult female profile has been drawn up and clinically approved. These various tools will be presented in Part 3 of this book.

Some women report that they have consulted a variety of professional and health services without being able to gain a clear diagnosis or any explanation as to their personality traits. This explains why it takes longer for women to conclude diagnostic tests for autism compared to their male counterparts who may receive a diagnosis at a much earlier age, often before or during school – the majority of women who come to consult with us are usually well into their 20s or older. Because the female profile of autism is generally less severe than that seen in boys, diagnosis is made later.

Habitually, a young girl with autistic traits and behavioural difficulties or aggression will be noticed early in her development by her parents or teachers. By contrast, the majority of young autistic girls are rather shy and reserved, and seek out little social attention. This explains the delay in recognition of the diagnosis. Several co-morbidities (or linked diagnoses) can be combined with autism. These are often the entry point into assessment or psychological or psychiatric services. As the classic approaches don't work optimally for autistic people (which is the case for medication as well as therapy), autistic traits must be taken into account so that women can be given the right guidance.

FRIENDSHIPS

The social aspect is central to the autistic profile. Challenges with social skills are frequently reported from a young age. Rules and social conventions are misunderstood, which contribute to feelings of ineptitude. Autistic adults relate that they found it difficult to form and maintain friendships at a young age. Not knowing how to join in with the group, they often stayed away and isolated from others. The development of making and maintaining friendships and social skills, which seems so spontaneous and natural among neurotypical children, is a real challenge for autistic young people.

However, we have observed a difference in girls – they have more desire to form friendships, but don't know how. With boys, the need to form friendships and social relationships is generally less developed. This characteristic is important to know, because often a professional will eliminate a possible autism diagnosis by simply asking 'Have you got friends?' The autistic woman will frequently answer 'Yes' (but very few, and, above all, these are deep, not superficial, friendships). Sometimes, friends are those met at secondary or high school. It is, however, more difficult to establish new relationships the older you are.

THE PLACE OF PLAY

For a young autistic girl, play is also different. For example, she might play with dolls, but in a functional way: she might be their teacher, and the dolls are her pupils. Like a mini teacher, the girl goes into character. Some young girls say that they prefer boys' toys because they are more rational than some 'girls' toys', which aren't logical and require imagination to 'make believe'. LEGO®-style blocks or Playmobil®-style toys enable them to build houses, towns, etc. Sometimes the need for symmetry in construction toys is observed (order, colour, shape, etc.).

SPECIAL INTERESTS

Many young autistic girls like to explore nature, look at leaves, flowers or insects, or build themselves a den in the woods. What sets them apart from other girls is their attention to detail in their observation and contemplation of nature. This interest can become very intense, or enjoyed in a more limited way, at the expense of other comparable activities that are enjoyed by non-autistic girls.

In their developmental history, some young autistic girls tell of their passion for reading, drawing, learning words or working with numbers, and very intensely. In this way, they can spend many hours alone, absorbed in books or textbooks, without ever getting bored. Reading encyclopaedias can also give them the intense pleasure of discovery and accruing knowledge. Here, again, it is not so much that the field of interest itself is unusual, but more the intensity of it that makes it characteristic of autism. Compared to boys, who sometimes take a very early interest in, for example, the lives of the US presidents, or dinosaurs, or the history of a certain country – and in great detail – an autistic girl is different in the near-uniqueness of her special interest. Neurotypical girls also develop passions, but with a larger variety of activities or themes – with the main difference being the intensity of the interest. Young autistic girls tend to develop a special interest early on, or a series of special fields of interest. Because they spend so many hours at a given activity or special interest, it gives them the opportunity to develop their expertise. They are autodidacts who love to learn through reading (blogs, tutorials, websites, etc.), which may eventually provide some of them with their career (Cook and Garnett 2018).

Among autistic people, special interests can develop in four stages (Attwood 2008):

1. A particular aspect of the object (an eye-catching detail that becomes the field of interest)

2. The category of the object (transport, animals, electronics, cuddly toys, trinkets, etc.)

3. Complex or abstract fields of interest, such as history, geography, the sciences

4. Interest in a person, fantasy literature or multiple special interests.

Professor Attwood also states that, alongside the development of special interests among women and girls, several behavioural observations will determine the female profile. Regarding friendships, some autistic girls, easily influenced by others, are prepared to do anything to have any type of friends/friend relationship. As they have difficulty judging character (or describing the character or personality of another person) and in decoding other people's intentions, they can, unfortunately, find themselves in situations of victimization and all kinds of abuse. Since their diagnostic characteristics are less visible (at the extreme end of the autism spectrum), they can pass undetected for many years. Because they have strategies to compensate for this socially, many women will appear perfectly well adapted, but this can all weigh heavily and become exhausting as the years go by. This can often lead to co-morbidities such as professional burnout, depression, anxiety or other physical health problems, etc. It is often a breakdown, after living so many years not being happy or comfortable in their skin, that leads women to seek out an assessment.

IMITATING SOCIAL BEHAVIOURS

Quite naturally, autistic girls navigate through or learn social skills by observing and imitating, in order to copy the social behaviours of other, more popular, girls. So on the outside they may seem perfectly socially adept, but this is as a result of the strategies they have put into place. What is more, autistic women and girls are by nature more sociable than their male counterparts, and they generally hope to form at least one meaningful friendship. Yet lengthy social or group situations will provoke anxiety and severe fatigue. This is why, at times, they need to retreat into their 'bubble' and recharge their batteries. This is what an autistic woman told me in an interview:

During family meals, and particularly when extended family came to visit, I would hide in my wardrobe as soon as I could. I had kitted it out with books, food, blankets, and I was very happy like that in my cocoon, never tiring of my books. My parents knew where I was... I needed to withdraw because there was too much noise, multiple simultaneous conversations, cooking smells... The sensory and social overload exhausted me. Alone, but never isolated, I went to the world I had created, with my characters, my stories, and I didn't feel the time passing.

For many, fiction can help them understand emotions and social behaviour. Through stories, films and sitcoms, they can learn to decode relationships. This is just one reason why they can spend hours reading and then re-reading novels, or re-watching films on loop – to dissect and learn social scripts.

PEER SUPPORT

Another way of learning how to develop socially and navigate social situations is with the help of a supportive peer or a trusted friend who can offer guidance and a sense of security. This friend becomes a point of reference. Liane Holliday Willey broaches this idea in her book *Pretending to Be Normal: Living with Asperger's Syndrome* (1999). She herself was able to survive nights out and college parties with the help of a trusted friend who would explain how to act, who to talk to, how to avoid problems, and so on. This sort of 'social translation' can clearly warn against a variety of mistakes as well as help avoid getting into difficulties. In adulthood, partners often take on this role. This 'translation' by a partner can help an autistic woman protect herself from risky situations and people with bad intentions.

A PROLIFIC IMAGINATION

An active imagination is another characteristic often found in the female profile. Many autistic girls have an imaginary friend, or invent an imaginary world. There are several reasons for this – to make up for a lack of real-life friends, for fun or for comfort and reassurance. An autistic girl may invent a female friend for herself with whom she will maintain an internal dialogue. This is what one woman told me in an interview:

Every Friday at the end of the school day, the other pupils would discuss their plans for the weekend. For my part, as I always did the same thing (read books), I had nothing to tell. So, I invented a friend, who was Asian, with whom I could explore (in my imagination) one of my other special interests: Japan. Thanks to him, I could eat typical Japanese dishes, read manga, look at maps of Japanese cities, and learn Japanese. This way, I could tell the others what I had been busy with during the holidays.

Another function of the imaginary friend is someone to recount the social events of the day to, in order to make sense of them. Sometimes, even verbally, an autistic girl will use examples from what she experienced that day, what she said and what she understood in her imagination, because that enables her to absorb her experiences in a logical way. This drive for the imaginary can even take her as far as adopting a new personality or changing her name. By becoming a new person, she can gain access to a new social role, sometimes inspired by or copying another girl who possesses these skills and a greater social capital.

These different coping strategies – social avoidance, copying, seeking peer support or masking – are therefore indicative of the social difficulties typically experienced by autistic girls and women. However, they can also be a way of showing interest in and an openness to other people.

An additional interesting point is that many books that have been published on the female profile are autobiographies. Many autistic women show a remarkable capacity for introspection. This enriches the understanding of professionals and clinicians, who, in reading them, can see what autism looks like from the inside.

CHAPTER 4

The Most Common Features of Autism

CAMOUFLAGING OR MASKING

During clinical interviews, many women talk about using social camouflaging as a coping strategy, masking their autistic traits in social settings. From a young age, girls adopt a series of behaviours intended to hide or compensate for their difficulties, and this often acts as a screen or mask. From that point on, they seem socially well adapted from the outside, but on the inside, it is quite a different story. As stated in Chapter 3, autistic girls and women are generally more invested in socializing and having meaningful friendship connections compared to autistic boys or men. Furthermore, expectations and societal pressure are greater, which leads them to adopt social masking.

These skills are learned. Simon Baron-Cohen, psychologist and researcher at the University of Cambridge, has co-authored two interesting articles on this subject (Hull *et al.* 2018; Rynkiewicz *et al.* 2016). Together with his colleagues, he has devised a questionnaire that assesses masking among autistic women. He describes three types of strategies: compensation, masking and assimilation. Table 4.1 shows some examples.

The self-observation Camouflaging Autistic Traits Questionnaire (CAT-Q) consists of 25 questions based on self-observations reported in the article by Hull *et al.* (2018). Ninety-two adults participated in the first study, and 354 adults took part in validating the questionnaire. The results confirm a link between maintaining a number of masking strategies, depression and anxiety. Moreover, women use more of these strategies than men.

Table 4.1: Examples of strategies

Strategy	Examples
Compensation	• Learning the social codes and conventions by studying books on the subject • Repeating behaviours seen in films, television shows or sitcoms • Using social routines and pre-prepared scripts (preparing a subject before a meeting, always saying the same thing when meeting a new person, practising polite phrases or social conversations when arriving at the office, with family or among colleagues)
Masking	• Making an effort to maintain eye contact • Paying attention to posture and gesticulation • Being vigilant with facial expressions • Adopting a relaxed expression or posture
Assimilation	• Avoiding social situations • Imitating other people's behaviour and attitude in different contexts (at an oral presentation or during a work project, at a family meal, etc.) • Giving a performance as if acting on the stage – playing a role as somebody else • Pretending to be like other people (Holliday Willey 2014)

Lai and Baron-Cohen (2015) underscore the importance of exploring the female profile in their article on the 'lost generation', which refers to the many women who have had a difficult route to obtaining a diagnosis. Far from wanting to label them or trying to describe a profile unique to autism, the aim is to increase understanding of their characteristics, encouraging self-acceptance and improving access to tailored services. Several of the participants in the study by Wiskerke, Stern and Igelström (2018) confirmed that it is preferable to obtain a diagnosis for a number of reasons, including getting a better understanding of their own characteristics. Moreover, they would like to raise awareness among the general public given the greater acceptance and tolerance of symptoms linked with autism.

Camouflage is used as a strategy for hiding or limiting stimming behaviours and involuntary movements. Wiskerke, Stern and Igelström (2018) explore the three different methods used by autistic women and transgender women in relation to this: substitution, isolation and active suppression:

- Substitution involves replacing a gesture or movement with a more subtle or socially acceptable alternative (playing with objects concealed in a pocket, fiddling with your phone, wriggling your toes inside your shoes, etc.). Although this type of movement is not seen exclusively in autism, it is involuntary and uncontrollable for autistic girls and women.

- Isolation involves withdrawing to a private place to allow the repetitive movements to take over or 'stimming' (walking in a circle, flapping arms, swaying, etc.). Several women who took part in the study confirmed that they hid away in their rooms from a young age to be able to indulge in a variety of stimming behaviours, which were enjoyable and helped them self-regulate.

- Active suppression consists of consciously stopping the movement. This strategy is linked to a fear of negative judgement and the fear of seeming odd. Autistic women who use this sort of camouflage maintain that they want, above all, to avoid any kind of attention.

In conclusion, Wiskerke *et al.* (2018) report that the negative impact of camouflaging stimming or involuntary movements is due to the non-acceptance of difference and the critical perception neurotypical people have of autistic people. And that the latter would like their differences to be accepted with a more constructive understanding of this form of expression and self-regulation.

TO FIND OUT MORE

In their article on the female profile, Adeline Lacroix and Fabienne Cazalis (2017) also address the idea of camouflage by referring readers to the graphic novel *Invisible Differences* by Julie Dachez (2020) This gentle, inspirational book follows the progress of a young woman through her daily life, and the traps she navigates that will eventually lead to her diagnosis. This work is highly recommended as a way of broaching the possibility of a diagnosis, or for constructively explaining the female profile.

In this way, this range of camouflaging strategies can work for several years, before exhaustion sets in as a result of the energy expended on keeping it up. At this point, a questioning of identity will follow. Who am I – behind the mask?

FEELINGS OF IDENTITY

Identity and self-esteem are closely interlinked. Since many autistic women and girls resort to camouflaging strategies, they can call into question their feelings of identity or sense of self. As a result of 'pretending' to be like others or adapting to expectations, they can lose sight of who they really are. One of the exercises put forward by the contributors in James Overholser's article (1996) aimed to improve self-esteem among autistic girls and women by asking them to compile a list of their qualities and their skills in order to give them a better balance of the elements that make up their self-esteem. This activity can also be carried out using five axes for guided reflection, inspired by Overholser, a cognitive-behavioural psychologist. Self-esteem is a multifaceted concept organized around four key axes (to adapt Overholser's work to the autistic context, we have added a fifth axis):

1. My academic and professional achievements, my hobbies, my special interests

2. My health and physical appearance

3. My interpersonal relationships (contacts, friends, etc.)

4. My emotional and family life, my marriage or long-term relationship

5. My knowledge and acceptance of my autism diagnosis.

For each of these, an evaluation of success is given as a percentage. Then it is a case of deciding which element deserves further exploration, and tailoring a structured intervention plan with clear objectives and positive strategies. Subsequently, the factors and behaviours that damage the development and maintenance of self-esteem must be broached.

To this end, Worksheet 1 presents an example of a worksheet devised by Danielle Paradis, consultant at Clinique Autisme & Asperger de Montréal.

✱

WORKSHEET 1: BEHAVIOURS DAMAGING TO SELF-ESTEEM

Thinking in 'black and white'
Thinking in absolute terms, such as using the expressions 'always', 'every time', 'never', 'there's no other way', etc. There are no half-measures.

For example, you think that you will never do anything good, that it will never work.

Strategy: *Think of other, similar situations, in which you succeeded. What skills and what strategies did you use?*

. . . .

. . . .

. . . .

Here's another example: If your performance is not completely perfect, you think you have totally failed.

Strategy: *What is your usual level of expectation? Did you have increased performance anxiety?*

. . . .

. . . .

. . . .

Excessive generalization
A tendency to overgeneralize certain difficult experiences. Jumping to conclusions based on partial information. Ignoring other, more positive experiences, which led to success.

For example, a single negative event can be conceived as the end of it, or, just because one thing goes wrong, you think it's all gone wrong.

Strategy: *Write a list of the events that are going well in your life, and which you feel happy about.*

. . . .

. . . .

. . . .

45

Mental filtering

An inability to see the positive side of an experience owing to a tendency to focus on the negative. Seeing the world in such a way that filters out any positive thoughts and events.

For example, you focus exclusively on one negative detail from your day, and you think the whole day is ruined.

Strategy: *Take the time to review the events of the day and evaluate what happened more objectively. Give yourself a moment to recharge your batteries.*

. . . .

. . . .

. . . .

Hasty conclusions

Drawing a hasty conclusion. Believing that you know what someone is thinking, or what will happen in the future, even if you can't read somebody's thoughts or see into the future. Having difficulties decoding other people's intentions; you can interpret other people's gestures and words negatively even if you don't have proof or the facts (this is linked to the theory of mind interpretation of autism).

Strategy: *Check with the person what you think you've understood. 'Have I understood correctly that...' or 'Please could you tell me more about that?'*

. . . .

. . . .

. . . .

Overdramatization and minimization

Overdramatizing or minimizing a situation so that it no longer matches objective reality. Regularly getting worked up about something of little importance. For people with depression, negative aspects are often exaggerated and positive aspects are underestimated.

Strategy: *Write a list of pros and cons, making an effort to balance out the two columns to help change the false, negative perceptions. For example: 'She succeeds; she is brilliant, while I never manage to finish a job' or 'If I succeed, it's down to luck; I had nothing to do with it'.*

. . . .

. . . .

. . . .

Catastrophic thinking

Always expecting the worst, even if that's unlikely.

Strategy: *Describe the situation objectively, define your emotion and make a note of the facts that prove that you are right to expect the worst, and the facts that prove the opposite.*

. . . .

. . . .

. . . .

Mental rigidity

Having thought patterns that indicate the way things 'should be' rather than considering the actual situation. The individual is confronted with their own inflexible rules. According to them, regardless of the circumstances, they should always say or do things in a certain way.

For example, you think you always have to pay attention.

Here is another example, this time relating to another person. You think she should have apologized. When you believe that the other person 'should' do or say something, this can make you feel angry, frustrated or resentful and, by the same token, can raise your anxiety levels.

Strategy: *What could you put in place to manage your anxiety better? How can you become more attentive to your thought patterns? How can you manage your own expectations?*

. . . .

. . . .

. . . .

. . . .

DEALING WITH EMOTIONS

Work on managing emotions will help tackle difficulties linked to mood disorders. Depression and anxiety are the primary co-morbidities observed.

If an autistic woman becomes overwhelmed with the intensity of her own emotions or equally the fatigue from interpreting the emotions of others, this may lead to meltdowns and perceived inflexibility in order to remain in a zone of known comfort. Often autistic women describe that although they can see the image of it in their mind, they find difficulty in describing the emotion or how they feel. This could potentially lead to reactive behaviour, which can negatively impact themselves or those around them. They may tend to react rather than reflect, which might result in rigid or problematic behaviours and attitudes. For difficulty managing emotions or emotive situations, a cognitive-behavioural intervention to help regulate and express emotion is recommended (Attwood, 2005a; Attwood and Garnett 2013a).

Considering oral linguistic expression and social expression may potentially be problematic, writing can be a constructive alternative means of communication. The important thing is to use all possible means to encourage emotional expression.

Concerning interpersonal relationships, a useful piece of advice is to find people who have shared special interests. This makes it possible to build trust and form long-term relationship with others. The main goal is to teach recognition and understanding of a variety of emotions so that these women feel capable of expressing just how they feel. Between joy and anger there is a whole range of feelings to discover. Emotional rigidity limits our experience and our self-expression. The concept of emotional intelligence neatly summarizes this targeted learning: recognizing your own emotions; managing them well, so that they are appropriate for the context; recognizing other people's emotions and interacting well in interpersonal relationships.

Some autistic women have explicit 'technical' knowledge related to the perception and understanding of emotions, but its implicit assimilation through experience seem to be generally lacking. This is illustrated by a tendency to overfocus on a particular region of the face compared to neurotypical people (e.g. the mouth instead of the eyes), which impairs their ability to process emotional expression efficiently. Follow-up interventions would need to focus on essential takeaways, in order to reduce the information overload that comes with explicit rather than implicit 'automatic' decoding of facial or non-verbal expressions of emotions.

At the brain level, results of several neuroimaging studies on this subject (e.g. Kana *et al.* 2011; Wicker *et al.* 2008) have revealed differences in amygdala activity and other regions of the 'social brain' in autistic people during emotion processing. Instead, studies reported activation of brain regions involved in executive tasks during social or emotional processing, as well as decreased connectivity between brain regions, meaning an intact ability to perceive emotional expressions, but an alternative cognitive strategy to interpret the perceived expression (Wicker *et al.* 2008). Overall, this suggests that autistic individuals may need to explicitly process emotions and social signals, leading to fatigue and stress.

To compensate for these difficulties, several learning activities or programmes are useful, such as:

- The Transporters, an animated series by Simon Baron-Cohen, Ofer Golan and Emma Ashwin (2009)

- Exploring Feelings program (Attwood 2005a)

- The Cognitive Affective Training-Kit (CAT-KIT) (Attwood, Callesen and Møller Nielsen 2006).

These are all aimed at improving recognition and emotional expression in young girls and teenagers. They provide clear learning outcomes, such as reading emotions in glances, exploring and dealing with emotions, and recognizing body language linked to changes of emotional state.

TO FIND OUT MORE

With the help of illustrations, photos and role-playing exercises, ask the autistic individual/person to run through the emotions, imitate facial expressions and identify situations (and scenarios linked to a range of emotions). The client also has to explore how their emotions fluctuate across the day (on a graded schedule) and keep track of how intense the emotions are, based on the idea of a thermometer. Once this has been accomplished, the more difficult emotions (anger, sadness, frustration and anxiety) are then addressed using a 'toolbox', a concept described by Attwood (2005a). This consists of a series of physical and relaxation activities, social encounters and positive thoughts (antidotes) that are recorded in a notebook. During role-play exercises, the client learns the sequence for managing the feelings by naming the emotion (or combination of emotions), and then uses the components of their toolbox, before reassessing the intensity of their emotional state now that they have more control over it. The aim is to reflect on emotions, name them and then manage them effectively. Otherwise, they risk expressing their emotions inadequately due to their intensity. This tangible learning outcome will help the client move to the next stage, which includes more advanced skills such as empathy, consent and emotional communication.

EATING DISORDERS

Anorexia is another condition linked to autism, especially in women. The root cause of anorexia and other eating disorders among autistic people has to be looked at from a number of angles. Sensory issues such as food texture, smell and taste are key here, as well as the swallowing reflex, which can be affected. Some autistic women cannot physically swallow or ingest certain foods, which can sometimes lead to a severely restricted diet and malnourishment. In other cases, obsessively counting calories and nutrients can contribute to the development of anorexia. If obsessive-compulsive disorder (OCD) is added to the clinical picture, the risks grow. Behavioural rigidity can also lead to anorexia. Some autistic girls and women are anxious by nature. They are not able to control external stress factors, like school, family relationships, performance anxiety or sensory overload. In an attempt to regain control, they may fixate on their food intake and body weight. Contrary to some hypotheses, most autistic girls and women do not have anorexia due to body dysmorphia, wanting to look more slim or a resulting lack of confidence.

Nancy Zucker's work (2015) lays out the similarities between autism and anorexia. She estimates that 5 to 10 per cent of people with anorexia are autistic women.

The following characteristics are given as contributing factors:

- Difficulty making friends

- Difficulty maintaining social connections, leading to a social withdrawal that persists among anorexic people, even after a return to a normal weight

- Rigid thought patterns and behaviours, with a need to keep things the same and a resistance to change

- Difficulty changing tack and a fixation on the detail rather than the bigger picture

- The presence of excessive anxiety.

In a letter to *The British Journal of Psychiatry*, Christopher Gillberg (2018) addressed the co-occurrence of autism and anorexia. The treatment of eating disorders should therefore be adapted to the autism spectrum disorder profile, as defined by several authors (Stewart *et al.* 2017; Westwood and Tchanturia 2017). A combination of educational, cognitive-behavioural and occupational-therapeutic approaches is recommended. Furthermore, the notion of control can be acquired with the help of strategies encouraging interaction and active participation.

TO FIND OUT MORE

The book *Hunger for Understanding* by Alison Eivors and Sophie Nesbitt (2005) has some interesting suggestions for encouraging interaction and active participation for autistic people.

CHAPTER 5

Sexuality: How Does Puberty Progress, and What Is the Sexual Profile?

Sexuality is a topic that has provoked a lot of interest in the current scientific literature. Generally, autistic people show the same interests and sexual needs as the neurotypical population, but outward signs and behaviours differ. Their lack of social skills and communication difficulties combine with obstacles to the establishment of interpersonal, sexually satisfying relationships.

In recent years we have seen a growth in theories and intervention models linked to autism and sexuality. Topics surrounding interpersonal relationships and sexuality are among those that retain the attention of families, professionals and autistic people themselves. The definition of sexuality is broad, covering love, intimacy, communication, emotions, experiences, social skills and behaviours. In order to understand and to intervene effectively for autistic people, it is essential to approach sexuality in all its complexity. This chapter will discuss current thinking, the socio-sexual profile of autistic women, and requirements for the teaching of social and sexual skills.

SEXUAL DEVELOPMENT AND PUBERTY

Several authors (Aston 2014; Gray, Ruble and Dalrymple 1996; Haracopos and Pedersen 1999; Hellemans and Deboutte 2002; Hénault 2005) argue for the existence of a distinct sexual profile among autistic people.

Puberty starts for girls with the menarche, or first menstrual cycle, which indicates the maturity of the reproductive system. Daily personal hygiene is recommended, since the surge in hormones leads to secretions (from the genital area, armpits, hair and face) and causes more intense body odour during puberty. It is worth remembering hypersensitivities to hot water, soap (both texture and fragrance) and the texture of towels and other linen, as all these aspects may be felt to be intrusive by some girls.

On a sexual and interpersonal level, breast development can provoke different reactions in different autistic girls. Since it is a visible change, some will be glad of the transformation, as a visible sign of puberty. But breast development can also be anxiety-inducing, which may entail reactive behaviours by the same token. It is important to approach changes by using descriptive visual information in order to reassure girls.

For some autistic women, vaginal penetration can be painful due to tactile hypersensitivity. This pain is comparable to that felt by women with vulvar vestibulitis syndrome (dyspareunia), with symptoms such as a burning pain at the vaginal opening. Treatment for vulvar vestibulitis includes some preventive measures aimed at rebalancing vaginal flora, and so avoiding irritations or infections among women who have shown a sensitivity.

TO FIND OUT MORE

The book *Asperger's Syndrome and Sexuality: From Adolescence through Adulthood* (Hénault 2005) details strategies to reduce the symptoms of vulvar vestibulitis in order to help understand genital sexual problems and the repercussions of sensory sensitivities on a sexual level.

SEXUAL EXPERIENCE

To learn more about the aspects of sexuality and sexual functioning in autistic people, a survey was carried out among 131 autistic adults (88 men and 43 women) from Canada, Australia, the USA, Denmark and France (Hénault and Attwood 2002). The study resulted in an increased understanding of the development, behaviours, emotions and sexual experiences and the role of sex in the lives of autistic people.

The Derogatis Sexual Functioning Inventory (DSFI) (Derogatis and Melisaratos 1982) considered 11 aspects of sexuality (desire, behaviours, experiences, self-image, etc.). The results from autistic respondents were compared against the norm of the wider population, and demonstrate little sexual experience among autistic people. An interest in sex developed on average at the age of 14, but first sexual experiences occurred at the age of 22 for the majority of autistic people. Of the 131 respondents, nine were virgins at the time they completed the questionnaire (Hénault and Attwood 2002). The low level of experience that was reported was accompanied by psychological difficulties and physiological manifestations such as nerves, loneliness or fear. The level of general knowledge about sexuality was lower than that of the wider adult population, despite a reported curiosity about sex.

Furthermore, it appears that autistic people's sexual needs are being fulfilled by a rich and diverse inner life, which contradicts the idea we sometimes hear that autistic people have a poor or non-existent imagination. On the contrary, the study's participants spoke freely about their fantasies, which were founded on sexual diversity and freedom from social constraints and taboos. They were in tune with their own sexual role and its characteristics. They were open-minded, and more attuned to their own values than to societal norms. This proves that there is a non-gendered sexuality and identity independent from social criteria of gender and sex. The results of this study have embedded important clinical knowledge.

THE INTERNET AND SOCIAL NETWORKS

Another reality must be taken into account since the advent of social media and the internet. Since many autistic people take an interest in computers and the internet, it is important to consider the reality of websites that hold millions of files with sexual, erotic and pornographic content. Parental and professional guidance is essential. Poor judgement, literal thinking and the risk of becoming overwhelmed when faced with illegal pornographic material is a constant problem. Likewise, visual stimulation accompanied by masturbatory behaviours can lead to a behavioural chain – in other words, a series of behaviours that have become associated over time and by routine (and often by ritual), and that can be difficult to break. The risk of developing a special interest, sexual obsession or compulsion is often linked to the consumption of pornographic material on the internet.

Also, online discussion sessions and dating apps often attract predators (Carnes, Delmonico and Griffin 2007; Edmonds and Worton 2005). As autistic people are more vulnerable on a sexual and inter-personal level, several rules ought to be clearly explained to provide them with a certain level of safety. Equally, supervision and instruction are recommended. In *The Asperger Love Guide*, Genevieve Edmonds and Dean Worton (2005) compile a list of recommendations for using the internet. For example, supervision by a parent or a peer will help the autistic individual understand and respect the rules while using social media or chatrooms and improve overall safety. By nature, more naive autistic people are at risk of venturing online incautiously, which is how predators can locate them and abuse their trust. According to guidelines taught by several sex education programmes (Hénault 2005; Hendrickx 2008), all online exchanges of a sexual nature should be avoided (words, intentions, photos, videos). Moreover, it is not recommended for anyone who is autistic to meet with an individual (even a friend) contacted online, unless they are accompanied by a parent, a responsible friend or a healthcare professional. If the meeting is permitted, it must take place in a public space. Under no circumstances should personal information be divulged (e.g. name, address, phone number, bank account details or credit card) (Hendrickx 2008).

SEXUAL HISTORY

Sexual history is an element that bears heavily on sexual development. Sexual abuse is common (Griffiths *et al.* 2002). A low level of sexual awareness has a negative impact on the notion of consent in relation to sexual demands made of autistic people. A sexual history of abuse can foster poor sexual conduct, because the abused girl might start to replicate, by imitation, behaviours that she had been the victim of. This is why a teenage autistic girl who has suffered inappropriate genital touching might repeat it on another person, since she cannot work out how intimate this behaviour is: she is only copying. This factor must be taken into consideration before embarking on sex education activities. In such circumstances, autistic girls would benefit more from individualized interventions, tailored to their own reality. Therapy in psychology and sexology is recommended.

VULNERABILITY TO SEXUAL AGGRESSION

Numerous studies show that potentially 90 per cent of autistic people have been, at some time or other in their life, sexually attacked or abused, and this is especially the case for autistic women and girls (Taillefer *et al.* 2015; Zeliadt 2018).

Several vulnerability factors can contribute to making autistic women and girls more susceptible to inappropriate sexual touching or sexual abuse, notably:

- Their problems with expressive communication

- The little credence they are given (when they retell the facts, they can unfortunately be disbelieved or their story rejected)

- Their lack of knowledge and education on sex

- Difficulties recognizing danger and reading the intentions of other people (theory of mind)

- Social isolation

- A lack of awareness of their right to refuse to submit to actions they don't wish to take part in (notion of consent).

Their level of maturity also influences sexuality. For many autistic people, there is a difference between their chronological age (their real age) and developmental age – a gap of several years. This gap affects their judgement. There may be numerous physical consequences to this, such as sexually transmitted infections or unwanted pregnancies.

There are also serious psychological and behavioural consequences, including depression, anxiety, regression to an earlier developmental stage, problems with interpersonal relationships, post-traumatic stress disorder (PTSD), low self-esteem, insomnia and sexual problems, to name but a few.

THE NOTION OF SEXUAL CONSENT

On the subject of consent, the complexities involved in giving and expressing consent, working out the other person's intentions and decoding their signals can cause confusion. During a consultation, an autistic girl recently asked me this: 'If a boy comes up to me, am I obliged to like him back? And if he wants to kiss me, or tell me he wants to be my boyfriend, do I have to want to, too?' She told me that she had met the student in one of her classes, who came to talk to her during breaks. He also invited her on a night out with friends. Then she added: 'But how am I meant to decode what he wants? Does he only want to talk about our class, or does he want to be my boyfriend or fall in love?'

It is worth looking more closely at courtship, the stages of a relationship and non-verbal communication. In this instance, with the help of scenarios, practical worksheets, videos and role-play, we were able to approach this topic using practical examples. Although it was impossible to find the exact same examples or identical elements as the autistic girl's situation, this young woman was able to build a repertoire of signals, sequences and meanings, and so she became better able to respond to the young man. By preparing the possible types of scenario, the young woman felt less anxious and could draw on a range of reference points.

Additionally, I recommend preparing some 'key phrases' for moments of hesitation. For example, if someone invites you out spontaneously, it is important to have some useful phrases prepared, such as 'I'll think about it' or 'I'll check my diary', to avoid feeling obliged to respond under pressure. To avoid uncomfortable situations and the risk of sexual abuse, it is important to understand how healthy relationships are formed, and how to avoid sexual abuse by setting boundaries and understanding consent.

SEXUAL EXPLORATION

High levels of sexual activity or exploration are sometimes observed among autistic women. This behaviour is expressed through an unrestricted exploration of sexuality. The deliberate search for sexual partners and experiences falls into the category of a special interest. During consultations, some women explain this by separating sexuality from interpersonal relationships. This dichotomy enables the occasionally intense exploration of different unconstrained sexual practices in an exploratory and curious setting. Some of them also describe a divide between their body and their feelings. 'My body is only instrumental. It's been imposed on me. I don't really live in it,' a young woman in her 20s once told me. 'Sex lets me feel my own body through pleasure, touch, pressure, but it's got nothing to do with love.' Clinicians report this sort of practice, too, but more research is needed in this area.

During an interview an autistic woman explained her experience and her perception of sexuality to me:

> It's only by following the 'sexual script' and routines that I can feel competent. I manage to replicate all the movements, as if in a scenario, so I take on a role often appreciated by my partners, as well as feeling more in control. On the other hand, I don't know how act in a relationship.

It is essential to inform and guide autistic women who are dating or interested in casual sexual relationships about the potential dangers, possibility of sexual abuse or finding themselves in situations they hadn't anticipated or imagined. Their deficit in relation to theory of mind (capacity to imagine the thoughts, emotions and intentions of the other person) risks limiting their ability to predict outcomes and can provoke misinterpretations, even leading to potentially dangerous situations, so providing guidance and information on consent is essential.

GENDER IDENTITY

Another component of identity is that of gender. Gender is an internal experience that is known only to the person who experiences it – only they are able to identify and express it correctly. This relates to a sense of belonging and being at ease with one's biological body; however, it is important to note that not all people who are gender diverse feel a sense of unease in their bodies. Clinical observations and discussions in a group made up of adults presenting a diversity of gender expressions point to a possible correlation between autism spectrum condition and gender dysphoria (Israel and Tarver 1997). From our point of view, this isn't a disorder, but rather an expression of gender identity and diversity. Gender diversity is described by A Gender Agenda, a gender rights organization, as an:

> umbrella term that is used to describe gender identities that demonstrate a diversity of expression beyond the binary framework. For many gender diverse people, the concept of binary gender – having to choose to express yourself as male or female – is constraining. Some people would prefer to have the freedom to change from one gender to another, or not have a gender identity at all. Others just want to be able to openly defy or challenge more normalized concepts of gender.

For gender diverse people, their identity is about presenting something more outwardly authentic to the world, whether they understand themselves to be differently gendered, or have no gender at all.[1]

Whether in terms of clothing, personality traits and activities or
physical appearance, it is a non-conflictual lived reality, and many
autistic people describe it as 'gender neutrality'. Clinical experience
and research (Davidson and Tamas 2016; Jones *et al.* 2012; Kourti and
MacLeod 2018) show that a proportion of around 30–40 per cent of
autistic people identify as non-binary.

Expressing a different gender identity may be related to difficulties linked to identity, whereby some clients want to become another
person to 'erase' their autism . An autistic woman explained it to me:
'As I don't feel like other people, and I don't seem to find my place in
the world, I must be a man.' This very important aspect must be taken
into serious consideration if we are to support teenagers and adults.

To avoid the distress and impulsive decision making in relation
to transitioning, it is recommended to follow guidelines (Strang *et al.*
2018) to monitor decision making and provide adequate follow-up. The
role of the professional is to support the individual sympathetically
and to encourage access to adapted services. Autism must be taken
into account to carefully support gender transitions, as described by
Kourti (2021). A chapter on this subject can be found in *Supporting
Autistic Transgender and Non-Binary People* (Kourti 2021).

TO FIND OUT MORE

For more helpful information, *Gender Is Really Strange* by Teddy
G. Goetz is an expansive resource about the nuances of understanding gender diversity.

SEXUALITY

It is important to note that gender diversity is distinct from sexuality, and one's gender identity does not equate to sexual preference.
In terms of sexual desire and sexual orientation, one woman from
the Mutual Aid Group for Autistic Women in Canada reported the

1   https://genderrights.org.au/information-hub/what-is-gender-diversity

following: 'When I feel sexual desire, it's the person who attracts me, no matter their biological sex.' This was the start of long discussions on the subject of sexual orientation. In fact, about 30–40 per cent of autistic adults I have spoken to have told me that their desire doesn't relate to gender. This can be considered either as bisexuality, or pansexuality. It is important to note the language here, as there is currently a lot of discussion in the queer community about the functional differences between these two sexualities, and these can't be flattened in such an easy way. Regardless of your preferred term for this sexual identity, we are using the larger definition, which is attraction to another person.

SEX EDUCATION AND INTERVENTION

The teaching of social and interpersonal skills is highly beneficial. As well as improving the quality of the autistic person's social interactions, interventions and sexual education programmes can be useful to help integrate these new learned behaviours into their daily lives. Gray *et al.* (1996), Haracopos and Pedersen (1999) and Hellemans and Deboutte (2002) all agree in emphasizing the importance of this approach, and since publication there have been more initiatives in teaching sex education. The interest shown by participants, their parents and professionals working with autism confirms the importance of accessing practical, interactive material.

The socio-sexual programme put forward in *Asperger's Syndrome and Sexuality* (Hénault 2005) uses both individual and group interventions structured around emotional relationships and sexuality. Learning is facilitated by practical activities, scenarios and role-plays. Each theme is supplemented with visual material to ensure concepts will be understood and retained. This programme is aimed at teenagers and adults. It consists of 12 workshops, each based on a different theme, such as love and friendship, sexual behaviour, prevention of sexual abuse, emotions in the context of relationships and the prevention of sexually transmitted infections.

The subject of successful relationships is equally crucial to cover. The anatomy of relationships, the stages of dating and the elements making up love and friendship should also be taught. To counter models seen on film or television, which are often inappropriate or unrealistic, visual material (films, videos, scenarios, descriptive worksheets on model relationships) is used, and then discussed and taught to autistic girls. Over the last few years, a detailed list of educational websites, teaching videos and models has been expanded and published in *Asperger's Syndrome and Sexuality* (Hénault 2005). Without going so far as to impose a rigid model or recipe, it combines examples of interventions and adapted tools that act as guidance – guidance that would otherwise be absent because of a lack of social and relationship experience.

CHAPTER 6

Personal and Professional Relationships

ROMANTIC RELATIONSHIPS

The subject of relationships raises several questions about adjustments to be made between an autistic woman and her neurotypical partner. Similar questions are also raised in the context of a relationship between two autistic people. In a romantic relationship, the expression of autistic traits and behaviours varies depending on multiple factors, such as prior experience, whether the autism diagnosis has been revealed and accepted, levels of communication, support and motivation between partners, and their family situation.

For some autistic women, intimacy is a vague concept with little bearing on the real world. Not that they don't wish to have intimacy with a partner – but some have only minimal experience of interpersonal relationships. This lack of intimacy and reciprocity between partners is one of the main sources of discontent among couples who come to therapy. Sexual satisfaction (frequency and quality) is not a gauge of success in relationships. Neurotypical partners relay that their autistic partner assumes that satisfaction as a couple comes down to an active sex life. Sex is just one of the many components of intimacy. This 'real-world, tangible' interpretation of intimacy is not uncommon in the autistic profile.

TO FIND OUT MORE

Several books address the reality for autistic couples. *The Partner's Guide to Asperger Syndrome* (Moreno, Wheeler and Parkinson 2012), *Aspergers in Love* (Aston 2003) and *Loving Someone with*

Asperger's Syndrome (Ariel 2012) are informative for both professionals and couples.

Marital dynamics should be approached with the autistic profile in
mind. Autism can impact or affect relationships on a daily basis in a
variety of ways. For example, rigid thinking, special interests, rituals
and sensory sensitivities sometimes lead to the autistic partner making demands or requests that may seem unusual to their neurotypical
or neurodivergent partner. The other person will have to adjust to that
reality one way or another. As these are tendencies inherent to autism,
they cannot be hidden.

SHOWING AND EXPRESSING AFFECTION

Affection is also at the heart of our interpersonal and family relationships. Among neurotypical people this is demonstrated by gestures,
words and actions. Professor Tony Attwood and Michelle Garnett
(2013a) have devised a practical guide to help enhance emotional
expression with a partner (or family member, for instance) in a range
of relationship contexts. By means of real-world exercises and scenarios, models responding to the other person's need for affection
can be learned, and that includes the needs of children or siblings.
In return, the other person will feel appreciated, and there will be a
positive feedback loop. To do this, each person's emotional expression, preferences and ease with demonstrating affection in a variety of
ways (gestures, compliments, actions, etc.) must be taken into account.
This programme, which was first targeted at autistic children, can be
adapted for adults. Efficiency studies have confirmed its positive consequences for both the autistic person and the people around them.

Worksheet 2, which was adapted from the book *From Like to Love for
Young People with Asperger's Syndrome (Autism Spectrum Disorder)* (Attwood and Garnett 2013b), is aimed at improving understanding of the
concept of affection. Indeed, the authors designed the programme
specifically so that autistic people can adopt affectionate behaviour
and arouse emotional expression in return. It is equally important for
neurotypical partners to understand the way in which autistic people
may express affection differently, and learn to identify and appreciate
this affection as opposed to the onus being only on the autistic person
to express affection in a more neurotypical manner.

WORKSHEET 2: HOW DO I DEMONSTRATE AFFECTION?

- What can I say to someone I love? What affectionate words can I use?
- What can I do to show someone that I love them? What actions can I take?

In words: How do I express affection?

Kind words:. . . . .

Compliments:. . . . .

Admiration:. . . . .

Jokes:. . . . .

Encouragement:. . . . .

Appreciation:. . . . .

Friendship:. . . . .

In actions: How do I show affection?

Listening:. . . . .

Spending time together:. . . . .

Helping:. . . . .

Affectionate gestures:. . . . .

Task: Show affection:. . . . .

Describe the situation:. . . . .

With whom:. . . . .

What sort of affection is it: words, gestures, actions?

. . . .

How did the other person react? How did that make me feel?

. . . .

In follow-up consultations or therapy sessions with couples, the topics of emotional communication, scripting and sexual behaviour, as well as desire and empathy, are worth covering in relevant and accurate terms. The key ingredient in all these reflections and exercises is an engaged and supportive partner. A couple's desire for evolution and sharing with each other must go hand in hand with a therapeutic approach. The two partners must be motivated, because they are going to invest their time and energy if a healthy relationship where both partners feel supported and understood is to be achieved. The therapy goes beyond the sessions as follow-up reflection and exercises will be required during the week. This process of growth and development can be painful, especially for the autistic partner if it feels like a lot of change and they are comfortable in their own routine. Sex therapy will cover all aspects of sex and sexuality, and must, above all, be adapted to the autistic couple's own reality. This work can be labour-intensive, but the investment is worthwhile.

Worksheet 3, which was devised by Danielle Paradis, consultant at the Clinique Autisme & Asperger de Montréal, presents topics for discussion between a professional and a couple. These are intended to encourage each person to share their ideas, emotions and perceptions, so that both members of the couple can reflect, give their opinion and listen to the other person. The worksheet provides a framework for discussion, which is reassuring when emotional and relational communication are the subjects for discussion.

*

WORKSHEET 3: BUILDING HEALTHY RELATIONSHIPS

The prelude to a relationship

- Self-knowledge: who you are, likes and dislikes, values, expectations, what you want and why you want to be in a relationship

- Believe that you deserve to meet a wonderful partner (putting aside social criticism and isolation, and a negative self-image)

- It is important to make decisions based on what you want (whether to be in a relationship or not).

The ingredients of a romantic relationship

- Sharing and connecting with your partner (activities, thoughts, passions, experience, etc.)

- Taking care of the other person (being attentive, making them happy, respecting them, etc.)

- Support (with problems, with completing tasks, etc.)

- Communication (expectations, needs, desires, emotions, confiding, using 'I' when making statements, e.g. I feel, I think, I need)

- Love and affection (affectionate and loving gestures)

- Quality time (fun, relaxation, sharing happy moments)

- Respecting each other's differences.

The ingredients of a friendship relationship

- Sharing

- Support

- Communication

- Affection

- Quality time

- Respecting each other's differences.

*

The ingredients of a healthy friendship

- Activities (having interests in common)

- Support (confiding in them).

Trust will build gradually as you spend time together, which is as much the case with friendships as with a loving relationship. It is important to trust your intuition!

The advantages and challenges of being in a couple

Choices to make:

- Living separately?

- Living together?

Advantages:

- Sharing your passions, creations and discoveries on a daily basis

- Sharing pleasure and intimacy

- Sharing daily activities (tasks, interests, etc.)

- Sharing expenses

- Avoiding losing yourself completely in solitary routines and rigid thinking

- Being forced to get outside your comfort zone (rising to the challenge)

- Answering a need for affection, comfort and stability.

Challenges:

- Making compromises

- Communicating

- Sharing your physical space

- Trusting

- Building the capacity to show affection

- Managing and exploring sensory accommodations (hyper- and hyposensitivities).

FAMILY RELATIONSHIPS

Regarding family relationships, there are multiple dynamics at play depending on the presence of autistic symptoms in other members of the close or extended family. The latest research estimates the presence of a genetic or hereditary link in 83 per cent of autistic people (Sandin *et al.* 2017). The confirmation of a diagnosis for a child or sibling often leads undiagnosed autistic women to recognize the same characteristics in themselves, which then inspires them to read up on the subject to find out more. Some women mention a clear understanding between family members with autistic traits (understanding each other, acceptance of difference, capacity for introspection regarding attitudes and observed behaviours). However, in other cases, rigidity or a perceived lack of empathy in family members can lead to conflict. In interviews, it is not uncommon for autistic people to relate their childhood memories by evoking a particular family environment dictated by their father's or their mother's personality, which, in retrospect, seems to have some characteristics in common. When considering whether to suggest a formal assessment of parents or siblings and benefits of diagnosis versus the harm a diagnosis could cause, factors to take into account are the person's age, overall physical health and any sensitivity or prejudice towards the subject. If it is decided that a recommendation of formal assessment would be futile, it is recommended to provide information on autism together with websites and crib sheets, or to simply tell them about an autistic adult's journey. Without being confrontational, providing this information is useful and can open the door to future discussions.

PROFESSIONAL LIFE AND JOB-SEEKING

Job-seeking, job retention and workplace politics are also themes to be explored. Many autistic women have the skills to do a job well, but it remains fundamental for them to access help and accommodations. Masking is often used in professional settings and will lead to burnout. Organizations such as Auticonsult France et Québec[1] and Neuro Plus[2] offer services intended to improve accessibility and job retention. These two organizations show solidarity with and value the talents of

---

1   https://auticon.com/ca-fr
2   www.neuroplus.org

autistic adults, making the link between them and employers. There are a variety of similar organizations in the UK and the USA.

Here is a list of support and services offered that address a range of employment-related issues:

- Depending on the assessment of executive functions, adapt the support and encourage initiatives. For example:

  - CV and cover letter

  - Job-hunting (spreadsheet to track the job search and to follow-up)

  - An explanation of why you want the job (possible interview question)

  - Role-play to prepare for an interview.

- Recommended strategies are as follows:

  - Keep a logbook or journal of emotions

  - A diary to organize tasks

  - Training in interpersonal skills and teamwork

  - Conflict resolution (how to go about it)

  - Disclosing the diagnosis.

TO FIND OUT MORE

Free worksheets detailing the strategies listed here can be found in *Autism Working* (Garnett and Attwood 2021).

CHAPTER 7

Seeking a Diagnosis and Recognizing the Profile: Resources and Tools

MOVING TOWARDS A DIAGNOSIS

A range of backgrounds can lead towards screening (e.g. classroom observation or a family history). In the developmental history of autistic girls, it's not uncommon for a teacher to have noticed difficulties with friendships or conversations, particular interests, a more autodidactic style of learning, or difficulties controlling and expressing their emotions. There might also have been a diagnosis for someone else in the family (a sibling, parent or extended family member), and as the parents find out more about autism, they recognize the autistic traits in their daughter, too.

The media, blogs and associations such as Autistic Girls Network[1] or Autistic Women & Nonbinary Network (AWN)[2] have provided information and increased awareness of female autism. When they were younger, many autistic women received a diagnosis of anxiety, depression, bipolarity, borderline personality disorder, eating disorders, attention deficit disorder (with or without hyperactivity) and so on. These diagnoses can lead to a more advanced investigation into characteristics, signs and behaviours, since they can be co-occurrent diagnoses alongside autism.

A large portion of the clinical assessment will focus on an atypical developmental history. Some aspects linked to social, relational and

---

1   https://autisticgirlsnetwork.org/autistic-girls
2   https://awnnetwork.org

communication difficulties are explored through questionnaires and a discussion with the professional. The clinical assessment guide in Part 3 of this book describes these aspects in detail.

In certain cases, one or more instances of selective mutism are described. These may have been triggered by extreme social anxiety. This inability to communicate verbally becomes more common during adolescence, but some women report selective mutism in adulthood as well (Simone 2013). Sometimes it is the environment that triggers the selective mutism (in class, during an outing or group activity, etc.), while it never occurs at home. In addition, parents and teachers report rigid behaviour and social withdrawal. In their games, young autistic girls prefer to take the role of a 'mini teacher' or 'headteacher', and give orders and instructions rather than playing reciprocally with other children and their siblings. They can also show aggression and an immaturity in conflict resolution.

Among women, difficulties linked to academic progress and job-seeking, and those in the area of relationships, can push them to look for information on autism and seek a consultation with a view to a diagnostic assessment. Life transitions often increase anxiety, which in turn leads to characteristics and behaviours emerging that had previously been buried or camouflaged. More visible and observable, the traits linked to autism come back to the fore, just as they had been in past: stereotypies are observed, mannerisms, cognitive rigidity, a greater need to control one's environment, etc. In other cases, a child receives a diagnosis, which then throws a light on the mother's traits. Many women come to a consultation in this situation. Having received their child's diagnosis, they say: 'I see myself in my son [or daughter], but over the years I have learned to overcome or mask my traits.'

GRIDS AND QUESTIONNAIRES FOR DIAGNOSTIC ASSESSMENT

In 2011, Svenny Kopp and Christopher Gillberg published the Autism Spectrum Screening Questionnaire (ASSQ)-Revised Extended Version (ASSQ-REV). This first tailored tool enabled clinicians to formulate the basics of the female profile. Several questions from it are included in the clinical assessment guide to the female profile, which is presented in Part 3 of this book. Furthermore, Attwood, Garnett and Rykiewics (2011–17) have initialized two questionnaires that have also received clinical approval. The Girls' Questionnaire for Autism Syndrome (GQ-ASC, ages 5–12 and 13–18, 2013) was first conceived in order to establish the characteristics and symptoms of young and teenage girls.

These first grids led to the development of the Questionnaire for Autism Spectrum Conditions (Q-ASC) (Ormond *et al.* 2017). This questionnaire, which was conceived for girls aged 5–19, contains 57 questions based around nine elements: (1) behaviours typical of the gender; (2) the sensory aspect; (3) expected behaviours; (4) friendship and play; (5) social masking; (6) imagination; (7) mimicking; (8) talents; and (9) special interests. The clinical guidelines defined in Part 3 of this book will gather together the characteristics and questions that must be asked during the interview leading to an autism diagnosis for the woman or girl.

PROFILE RECOGNITION RESOURCES
FOR HEALTH PROFESSIONALS

The clinical assessment guide presented in Part 3 will cover the clinical characteristics of the female profile in their entirety, as well as detailing the diagnostic instruments that have been scientifically approved. This procedure, which has also received clinical approval, constitutes the basis of a diagnostic interview. The doctor or first-line healthcare professional (school psychologist, for instance) can use it as a starting point to explore the patient's characteristics with a view to referring her for formal assessment.

In her book *L'autisme apprivoisé*, Sandrine Lebrun (2015) explained diagnosis another way, describing the daily life of an autistic women through the eyes of her cat. Touching, gentle and intelligent, this book is a perfect companion to exploring or disclosing an autism diagnosis.

Disclosing a diagnosis to those around you is a major step. Many women wonder who they can talk to about their investigations, and how to talk about it.[3] This is, of course, linked to how open we are in different environments (whether family, school or in the workplace). As female autism is still fairly unknown, it is important to select the

---

3   Some websites are excellent sources of accurate information tailored to the female profile. See, for example, www.cjausome.ca/spectrum-women; www.autism.org.uk/advice-and-guidance/what-is-autism/autistic-women-and-girls; www.neurodiverging.com/2021-books-about-autistic-women; www.autismawareness.com.au/understanding-autism/women-girls

right person to talk to, to avoid stigmatization or outright denial. Even worse, some autistic women are told that they are looking for a diagnosis to find an excuse for the way they are, or because they are attention-seeking. Finally, we hope that this book will become a vector of knowledge and acceptance, and of benefit to many autistic women and girls!

IT'S RAINING ON MY DREAMS! BY ISABELLE QUEYROI-MALLET[4]

In the Year of Grace 2015...or should I say, in the Year of Disgrace 2015, on this cold autumn day, the Autism (Asperger's) diagnosis fell like a guillotine, severing all hope of fitting into the mold someday. I still remember the wild dance of leaves swirling everywhere, while it rained on my dreams. At least, on the dreams of grandeur and success that I had absorbed from my family, which had beautiful expectations for my future. Throughout my childhood, I was labelled as a mad scientist, "Tarzanette," or a prodigy, but the budding genius in me never found its meadow to flourish in. The reason, it seemed, was a curious and incurable ailment within me. There was indeed something in me that hindered the realization of my plans and instilled an extraordinary consideration for all intellectual things. And that was the question, indeed: the norms!

I clumsily and with such innocent candor got entangled in these invisible limits, and everyone forgave me for these politically incorrect deviations. "Zaza the Tarzanette," screaming deafening cries of silence in her zebra costume, swung from label to label: "the wild one; the crazy one; the asparagus." From the top of unattainable peaks, I cherished and preserved a submerged world, populated by fabulous animals and small, kind, loving, and joyful beings, singing under a white sun with enchanting melodies. There was an extraordinary peace and calmness in that uterine underworld, where all vibrated in idealized harmonies. And when I descended from my spheres, I lived the hell of a world I did not understand, imprisoned in an alabaster straitjacket destined to shape me differently than I was. Nicknames scarred my identity; the lashes of a backward education imprinted their refrain: "regain!" Soon, however, the dawn of renewal...

---

4   Please note that this section has not been edited; it is as the author wrote it.

The budding genius grew as best it could between the gray cobblestones of Paris. The sprouting of a stunted self between the mesh of the alabaster straitjacket had thwarted the perverse plans of the hostile universe that besieged me. As I laughed at the physical and psychic straitjackets worn alternately since forever, the rebel had to be tamed by sultry chemistry. And one day, the hurried footsteps of my mother on the pavement of Paname were as intense as her anticipated delight in seeing me confined among the mad! First encounter with a Pontiff of psychiatry who decided otherwise! After numerous tests, questioning, useless hesitations, without logic and against the pathogenic logos, he stamped me as "gifted"! My mother's bitter little world collapsed suddenly, tolling the bell for her ominous project. Since then, I had a relative peace with those close to me who gradually got used to this being that grew askew.

I grew unkempt and cantankerous, flourishing in my lifelong passions: writing, literature, theater, philosophy. The setting was too hideous, keeping me away from the Court of Loves. But it contained a flower with a thousand colors that perfumed words, enchanted concepts, and delighted astonished scholars.

In this grotesque mismatch, I limped through my life. I limped sometimes gauche and brainless, sometimes ugly and awkward. At that time, the gaze of others, however hurtful, did not affect me because I enjoyed the flair that suits the daring so well. I understood nothing of personal relationships. Yet, I had many friendly and intimate conquests. I understood social codes no better! But everyone came back to me as quickly as a boomerang, loving these candid awkwardnesses. Despite myself, I offered that unique little something with a taste of "come back for more" that excited the gourmet craving ambrosia. I conquered useless Everests and feasted on futile victories.

Then one day, tired of my deserted Eden, I flew to that white paradise filled with the richest promises. I left behind the ailing poet, the hungry artist in search of Matrie. I had an appointment in an unknown land...my promised land. Another one! Over the ocean, the chants of my little underground world rose to me, celebrating its new dawn and burying its Tarzanette. "Zaza the crazy one," "Zaza the wild one," "Zaza the genius" had hung up her vines to put on wind soles.

Bohemian Montreal welcomed me in the warmth of its eclecticism. I had finally found my meadow. Here, no one bruised me with their devastating gaze. Freely, I could be Quasimodo in majesty! I was breathless with happiness. But it was short-lived because, one December evening, I crashed on the frozen ground of my beloved city. A missed rendez-vous! I remember that the urban gray contrasted with the dance of joyful lights that illuminated the city in anticipation of its first Montreal Christmas. Christmas...symbolically considered a time of truce and miracles... I awaited mine. Despite the distance from the land of France, the past played tricks on my memory and galloped on the tortuous waters of the Atlantic to mock me better.

"Zaza the crazy one," "Zaza the genius," "Zaza the Tarzanette" was back! She settled back into this intruder that I had now become. The uterine world reappeared suddenly, sparkling with blinding lights, shouting thunderous songs that frightened the little fabulous animals. The cacophony of dissonant harmonies marked my diaphanous skin. But what was wrong!? New land but old ailment. I covered my ears, holding my breath to stifle my frantic reason.

And then one day, the pounding of my hurried steps on the cold pavement of Montreal. A taste of déjà vu! Suddenly, the maternal face in cellophane stretched into a victorious grimace. In the murmur of my questions, in the heaviness of my uncertainties, I beat the rhythm on the pavement of this new elsewhere. Now, mother to myself, I was in search of that asylum of the insane that was forever destined for me.

Another encounter with another Pontiff who declared an unabashed flame of admiration for the one so deeply buried, curled up in her pocket-sized cocoon. He stamped me with "Asperger." Another label...heavy to bear that one. Never did the gaze of others seem so deadly to me. Through their eyes, I became a living flaw, a hopeless anomaly that could not be repaired. I became a puzzle whose survival depended on a subtle assembly of pieces of grandeur weighed down by parasitic pieces, somewhat like a chess game... Am I just a chess piece all by myself!? Tossed from lands to lands at the foot of the trees of my wonderful universe, I wandered in sterile cognitive circumvolutions. Stranded on these desolate lands, once adorned with vermeil, the little beings watched me in silence. The stamp consumed me, relit me. The little fabulous animals melted into wandering clouds. Forever the feeling of missed appointments with the world, with others...it rained on their dreams! And on this blue October day, I had made the best of encounters: myself...and, in the salt of my tears, I was born again.

© Isabelle Queyroi-Mallet, November 2018

PART 2

STORY OF AN ADULT DIAGNOSIS

ANNYCK MARTIN

A note on language: Annyck's memoir refers to Asperger's syndrome, as it was the diagnosis she received at the time of her assessment and the term she used when she wrote the original version of this book several years ago. Today, she feels connected to the neurodiversity paradigm, which views diversity in human functioning as normal, valid and necessary. Neurodivergence includes autism, but encompasses other dimensions of human functioning, such as giftedness. She now identifies as a neurodivergent person and artist.

AUTISTIC GIRLS: A SILENT PROFILE

It took me several years to identify the characteristics that I function by. It is by means of observations and analyses that I arrived at the understanding I have of them today. Before that, I had noticed certain differences between my mode of functioning and that of most of the people around me. Nevertheless, as I was unaware that these characteristics are interrelated and that they have a common cause, I couldn't envisage them. They all seemed to me to be a pile of disparate pieces.

How do we talk about something we can't perceive or even conceptualize? How can we ask for help with difficulties we don't know the name for? Therapy I had pursued in the past was intended to help me feel more coherent. But how do we build a coherent identity when we remain ignorant about an entire portion of ourselves? And when that missing portion forms the basis of our functioning? Too often, autistic girls have 'flown under the radar'. And yet obtaining a diagnosis is to get hold of our instruction manual – and that can change lives.

My life has taken a turn for the better these last few years. I hope that this book that Isabelle and I have written will give all autistic girls, teenagers, women and people who relate to the characteristics of the female presentation the chance to improve their lives, and to see their suffering diminish or even disappear. You are not alone! No matter how old you are, getting to know and understand your functioning will open the door to new worlds, a new sense of balance, and new possibilities coming true.

In the chapters that follow, I refer to several professionals with whom I had contact: Jonas is psychologist #1, who brought me the subject of autism. Alice is psychologist #2, with whom I did psychotherapy a few years later. Sophie is the socio-professional counsellor I later refer to. Psychiatrist #1 (not named) is the person I consulted at the same time as my follow-up with Jonas, and who refused to give me a referral to go and do an evaluation in the public health system. Psychiatrist #2 (also not named) is the professional specializing in autism with whom I had a telephone conversation to try to access an evaluation in the public health system (which was not possible due to a moratorium and the impossibility of obtaining a referral from psychiatrist #1). For clarity and to aid the reading of my text, I decided to use the invented forenames Jonas, Alice and Sophie for the psychologists/socio-professional counsellors who saw me.

In recent years, the names in the field of autism have evolved as well as the way we understand autism, as more and more researchers now rely on participatory research that recognizes the experiential expertise of autistic people and addresses what is important for them in their lives as their preferences (and not just the perspective of parents or caregivers). In the same way, more and more autistic academics and researchers are revealing their neurodivergence and becoming openly involved in autism research, which allows us to question certain perceptions and

think differently about how to support autistic people throughout their lives. My vision of autism is close to that presented by
the paradigm of neurodiversity, which recognizes autism and
other forms of neurodiversity as normal varieties of human
function – in other words, the equivalent of biodiversity in
neurological form.

CHAPTER 8

A Spotlight on the Characteristics

TOO MUCH NOISE, MOVEMENT, SMELLS

I was 39, in 2011, when Jonas, a psychologist I was seeing for anxiety and health problems, asked me a question that took me by surprise. He asked me whether I thought I had any autistic traits. I had just shared with him a situation I was regularly experiencing and which I was struggling to cope with: when I find myself somewhere like a cafe or family gathering, where there is a lot of noise, movement and smells. I explained to him what that felt like to me.

In a situation like that, it is as though each one of my senses is suddenly excessively in demand, and my organism perceives everything too loudly, without being able to sift or triage the information it is receiving. The result is an intolerable tension that can only be calmed once the racket diminishes significantly, once the cacophony is over, or once I remove myself away from the situation that makes me feel so overwhelmed.

For a long time I blamed myself for having difficulties in settings like this, so incomprehensible I found the reactions they caused in me. I have always loved to observe, and I have noticed that the majority of people in similar circumstances seemed to be at ease, keeping control of their faculties and chatting with others, and enjoying it. Their capacity of being fully present and attentive seemed unaffected by the context, although I myself usually came away drained to the point of having to go for a lie down, and taking several days to replenish my energy by giving myself time alone at home. For a long time I tried to mask this problem, with alternately more or less success. I still find I want to hide it, at the same time by force of habit, by wanting to feel 'like everybody else' for a while, but also – and most of all – because it's difficult for me to translate these feelings, to manage to communicate them, their effects and their magnitude, to other people.

When I'm especially tired or unwell, my level of tolerance of stimuli is lower, and I can no longer stand it. During an episode like this, it is as though my nervous system has arrived at the end of its resources, and whatever I do, it collapses.

ITCHY LABELS AND FABRICS

During this session, Jonas asked me several other questions that I found surprising. Among other things, he asked me whether, as a child, I tolerated labels on my clothes. As a little girl, I couldn't stand any tags or labels in my clothes, and was very sensitive to the texture of certain fabrics. At the time of this discussion, I didn't know anybody else around me, as a child or later on, who had to systematically remove labels from their clothes to be able to wear them. It is typical of the sorts of details I learned early on to be quiet about, and which are scattered across my everyday life to this day.

SOCIAL CONTACTS

Jonas also reminded me of various anecdotes I had gradually shared with him concerning social contacts. After analysing them, I realized that it was a subject I had never considered explicitly in the follow-ups and support sessions I'd had.

For example, my transfer to the Cégep[1] was one of the times in my life I have felt most settled. This period is like a benchmark for me. It was the first time I felt competent navigating the social world. I was studying special education, and I was participating fully in student life. It was novel for me to feel part of a friendship group. Our little group included about 10 students, and I felt at home with them. I was seen as someone original and creative. The fact that it was in a living

---

1   The Cégep (general and professional teaching college) corresponds either to the end of general high school or technical college. This study programme is completed before university in Québec.

environment very open to differences probably contributed to how well integrated I was. A teacher I shared some creative affinities with was also a reference person who supported me during this time. Her support helped me to express myself better, and open myself up to other people, as well as helping me understand group situations. I am still grateful to her for this today.

During our discussions, Jonas took it upon himself to remind me of another aspect of my student life I'd told him about, and a subject I tended to avoid. During my college studies I lived in a student residence, and my nickname was 'the resident ghost'. In total I lived for four years in the halls of residence. For the first three years I didn't form a bond or maintain a connection with any other resident. But in the final year, the opposite happened. At the time, I was studying preliminary courses for university admission, and I no longer moved around with my classmates from the previous years. So I attended classes in ghost mode, while at the same time a close friend moved into the halls of residence and I started to mix more with other students who lived alongside me on campus.

This story is quite common among autistic people. Specialists tend to use the metaphor of filling a 'social bucket' to explain the difference in social needs between someone who is autistic compared to someone who is not:

> Some typical individuals have a large social bucket that can take some time to fill, while the autistic person has a small bucket, or cup, that reaches capacity relatively quickly. Conventional social occasions can last too long for someone that is autistic, especially as social success is achieved by intellectual effort rather than natural intuition. Socializing is exhausting. (Attwood 2008, p.91)

To sum up, once the maximum capacity of a day's social interactions has been reached, the surplus becomes 'too much'. The autistic person can keep up appearances for a certain length of time, but not beyond that. Social fatigue is generally more prevalent among autistic people than among those with a more typical functioning. This fatigue stems in large part from the fact that interactions with other people are carried out by means of an intellectual process rather than intuitively. This means that the autistic person has had to learn by observation, or formally, by reading or watching television programmes on the subject, how to start conversations and keep them going. Women and girls, in particular, more or less consciously train themselves to mask these aspects of their functioning in a variety of contexts. Thus, engaging with someone does not come easily or naturally, even to the more skilled among us.

Lucila Guerrero, artist, author and militant autist, whose trajectory is especially inspiring, describes her way of functioning during interactions with other people:

> During conversations, my brain is working hard to decode gestures and voice intonation, and analyse the context. When it comes to arguments, I need time to process the sense of phrases and respond, to make associations and find the right words. Sometimes, they don't come to me until the next day! (Guerrero 2013, p.33)

For many autistic people, finding themselves in a social situation sets into motion an array of action plans, so to do this an interior monologue is constantly at work behind the scenes. For me, it manifests itself in having to remind myself to say hello; to link the current conversation to our previous one by asking about some current work, or something else important to my interlocuter; to consider where I should stand within the group; to gauge eye contact, etc.

To make a comparison with my experience during the Cégep: I gave it all that I had to be able to interact socially in the daytime, in my lessons and breaktime. Once evening came, I had to withdraw and be in a quiet place where I could go about my business alone, in my room in the halls of residence, to replenish my energy. During my last year in the halls of residence, the place where I socialized was the opposite but the principle remained the same – in other words, an equivalent amount of time spent interacting or not interacting with other people in a single day.

GROUP SITUATIONS AND BULLYING

In practice, family and group situations are those I struggle most with. As a little girl, I spent most of the festive period in a cousin's bedroom, sitting on the floor in front of a shelf full of books. I preferred books to my cousins' games, which seemed too noisy and hectic to me. I was happy in the company of their books! Likewise, I then became a rather introverted teenager, spending most of my free time reading and drawing. At the end of one school year, a teacher wrote something to me which started like this: 'To Annyck, hidden behind her books'. Books were a refuge and provided an escape when compared with a harsh world in which I struggled to find my place.

Like many autistic people, I was bullied by other pupils at secondary school, mainly in the form of teasing and shoving. I bottled it all up, keeping a diary and writing poems instead. I can remember some very dark times. Adolescence is the time I truly became aware of the gaping chasm between myself and my peers. I quickly noticed the differences between my functioning and theirs. I just wasn't interested in the same things as them. I wasn't remotely interested in make-up kits received for Christmas. I couldn't fathom their infatuation with clothing brands, or see the point of paying more for something, like a jumper, bag or designer trainers, just because it had a favoured logo printed on it. Unlike my peers, I also had little interest in actors, singers or musicians of the time. I got into music, boys and fashion late, once I was a young adult.

As a teenager, I was mostly interested in books, human biology and arts and crafts. I loved – and still love! – learning, observing, analysing and thinking, or, as I like to put it, getting to grips with the hidden side of things, or the 'how it works'. By reading, drawing and writing, I tried to get to grips with the world around me, the people, the strange planet I'd landed on, to bring some order to what sometimes seemed to me like pure chaos.

CAMOUFLAGING: BOTH FREEDOM AND CONFINEMENT

Towards the end of secondary school, I noticed that when I masked my differences – such as my social difficulties, my preference for being alone and my academic abilities – the bullying got less, and even stopped. So I started to battle against who I really was deep inside. With considerable effort, I succeeded in making it all almost invisible from the outside, except in times of stress, tiredness or illness. The only downside was the strategies I'd had to put into place to achieve this. I'm referring to my methods of compensating, and their excessively high price. Basically, I had to amputate a fundamental part of myself to get there. This amputation was not without its consequences over the long term.

TO FIND OUT MORE

'Social camouflage' is a key theme in scientific works on the female profile of autism. See, for example, 'The experiences of late-diagnosed women with autism spectrum conditions: An investigation of the female autism phenotype' (Bargiela, Steward and Mandy 2016) and '"Putting on my best normal": Social camouflaging in adults with autism spectrum conditions' (Hull *et al.* 2017).

I ended up hating the girl inside me who struggled to engage with people, who didn't know where to stand or how to behave in a group context or in new situations. I was battling against a part of me that I associated with the suffering I had gone through at the hands of my classmates. In my heart of hearts, I felt broken, defective, and I was angry at myself. I had learned to hide these aspects of my personality in the hope of avoiding people attacking my sensitivities. In so doing, I also set about hiding these aspects from myself, which made my camouflage even more effective. This is probably the main reason why I never thought of speaking openly about the difficulties I'd had socially, before my psychologist raised the question. The idea of talking about it would never have occurred to me, given that I had stowed these aspects of my personality elsewhere, in 'another person'. Discussions with Jonas opened the way for me to progressively get back in touch with these dimensions, which I had put to one side.

A MODIFIED APPROACH

Other topics were raised in the course of these first discussions on the subject of autism. I remember that Jonas mentioned that he had had to modify his approach with me, since I didn't respond well to confrontation or other methods that are usually effective in therapy.[2] He connected my unusual reactions to the presence of autistic traits and

---

2   During a conversation with Isabelle, she told me that confrontation often causes shutdown, given that it increases anxiety and therefore cognitive rigidity among autistic people. On this subject, she mentioned Professor Tony Attwood's work on emotional regulation, as well as talking about the cognitive approach, which is interesting in that it seeks to increase cognitive flexibility.

said to me that if a prior diagnosis had been made, his approach would have been different from the start. Despite the time that's passed, I can't explain the differences he made to his approach, and I therefore don't have any tangible examples to give. The only thing I noticed, that coincided with the period he was referring to, was that I felt different during our sessions: I felt a lot less anxiety, pressure and tension during our meetings. I felt safer, which meant I went there with less apprehension, and this facilitated our discussions.

THE FIRST PIECES OF THE PUZZLE

Our first discussions on the subject of autism provoked contradictory reactions in me. Of the dominant reactions, I felt embarrassment, on the one hand, and curiosity, on the other. Embarrassment, because I felt I had been stripped naked, which made me feel uncomfortable. At the same time, I felt curious, because the points raised possessed a specificity, a colour that I recognized deep inside of me, and this made me want to explore this path in more depth.

In a logbook that I kept at the time of my therapy, I wrote that this first light-bulb moment seemed to gather together elements I had previously thought to be disparate, and which I had never thought could go together. The mental image I had then was one of an ultra-violet light that had come to bring certain objects from a batch to my attention and make them stand out from the undifferentiated lava in which they bathed. The new lighting allowed me to reveal links between these objects, to note their common nature, which brought me greater coherence and understanding of my inner world. Further on in my journal, I said that with this light I had the impression of perhaps holding in my hands all the pieces of the puzzle. It was a bit as though, until then, I had spent my life looking at a pile of random objects, never understanding how they went together, nor even the relationship between them.

This discovery filled the gaps in the knowledge I already had of myself, and which the story of my life couldn't explain on its own. I found this disconcerting and exciting all at the same time. I quite possibly had in my hands the start of an instruction manual that corresponded much more closely to the way I functioned than the every-day, normal instruction manuals I took note of all around me, none of which gave me what I needed to protect my well-being over the long term and live up to my potential. During these discussions, Jonas asked me to read up on the subject, which I willingly did.

TO FIND OUT MORE

I tell the story of some of the challenges I've overcome in my first book, *La crypte cassée: Essai sur l'écriture posttraumatique* (Martin 2010).

CHAPTER 9

A Journey in Reading

AN INITIATION INTO AUTISM

In the weeks that followed, I took Jonas's advice to read up on the subject. I started by going through general documents I had found on the internet. This preliminary reading helped me get to know the characteristics of autism and, more specifically, what was previously called Asperger's syndrome. It is a fascinating subject for anyone interested in human functioning. Since I was very young I have always been interested in human biology and psychology. This new research area naturally fitted in well with my other fields of interest.

I read a lot in a short time, and sorting through my readings was done quite quickly. I must admit that what I initially read left me doubtful. Descriptions taken from diagnostic manuals didn't seem to me sufficiently backed up to provide a full definition. Some aspects fitted me, but others, not so much. For example, I don't talk ad nauseam about subjects that interest me, as is seen in some autistic people. In fact, I speak very little about the subjects that spark a passion in me, apart from in very specific situations and with certain people, like a friend, a colleague or an open-minded person with whom I share some artistic, intellectual or other interests, and with whom I feel comfortable.

Later on, I read that, according to Professor Tony Attwood (2008), autistic adults are more inclined to read than speak about their special interests. This means that not everyone fits the mould of the autistic person who wants to share their interests with anyone who will listen. I also didn't think I had trouble reading the facial expressions of my interlocuters, as some books mentioned. When I shared this thought with Jonas, he told me that he had noted I had difficulty reading facial expressions more than once, and that this had, in fact, happened a few times during our discussions. His comment took me by surprise, since I perceived (and still perceive) any number of subtleties relating to other people's functioning. Sometimes, this oversensitive perception can become irritating and even overwhelming to me, as though I've got to the point of seeing 'too much'.

After some thought, I came to the conclusion that this apparent disparity between my perception and my psychologist's impression of it needed to be nuanced. I do, in fact, see a great deal of detail relating to other people's functioning, and I generally manage to build an accurate picture and a clear evaluation. Nevertheless, this clear-sightedness relies on particular contexts – that is, when I am in an 'observational position' or thinking 'with hindsight' after an interaction or encounter. As soon as I get involved actively in a conversation, it becomes more difficult for me to 'read' what is happening 'live'.

While some observations left me doubtful at first, other characteristics I had become aware of matched aspects of my functioning very closely. These features related, among other things, to the perceptive, sensory and social spheres. I found it startling how accurate the descriptions were. There were enough disparate fragments to make me keen to explore further.

I want to specify that, during my research, it was important to me to adopt a cautious and level-headed approach. I tackled the subject the same way I had tackled many other subjects that had attracted my attention over my lifetime. I am someone who takes pleasure in discovering and analysing things. I love expanding my knowledge on topics, and I try to do so by keeping an open, critical and reflective mind. When I embark on a process of study such as this, I do it rigorously. I am therefore careful to refer to a wide range of reputable and reliable sources in order to form more accurate ideas.

THREE BOOKS TO DELVE INTO

After this initial more generalized reading, I turned to more targeted books. The first was *Musique autiste: Vivre et composer avec le syndrome d'Asperger* (Ouellette 2018). This choice of reading came to me by happy accident. Around the same time as Jonas raised the possibility of autism at our meetings, the article 'Vivre et créer avec le syndrome d'Asperger' ['Living and creating with Asperger's syndrome'] (Martin 2011) was published in *Journal L'UQAM*, which I subscribed to.[1] The article briefly told the story of Antoine Ouellette, a musician running some courses at the university, who received a diagnosis of Asperger's syndrome at the age of 47. The article mentioned several characteristics present in people with Asperger's, such as frankness, authenticity and honesty. The text also indicated that people with Asperger's were more subject to anxiety, obsessions and social isolation. Several of these aspects fitted me.

I am not someone who indulges myself often, but when I do, when I'm feeling confident, or in my writing, I can be very transparent and authentic. In some situations, I can be quiet to protect myself, but I don't know how to play with masks or complicated social games (which I hate). On the subject of the challenges I have encountered along the way, one of the main reasons I went to therapy was that I had significant anxiety, which was difficult to manage in certain circumstances. As regards social isolation, I had lived in the same area for around 15 years and, rather like when I lived at the student halls of residence, I hardly knew anyone beyond my partner, our daughter and a few family members. The article described how Antoine had been a gifted and dedicated student, which was also the case for me. I was a child who had succeeded well in school without having to try and who went unnoticed in class. The article also mentioned Antoine's aversion to sport and that he had been the victim of bullying, two other points that matched my experience.

During my research, I also watched the video of a presentation by Antoine in a library in Montréal (Ouellette 2011). As I watched, I could see that his face wasn't in any way lacking in expression, and nor did he speak in monotone, two characteristics sometimes found in people with Asperger's. Overall, even if I could see he had a somewhat unique personality, his autism didn't exactly leap out at you. I saw that it was possible to be Asperger's without it being clearly visible. This realization was important to me, since my functioning is very much more interior than exterior.

---

1 Journal of news linked to the Université du Québec à Montréal (1974–2013). It has now been replaced by the website Actualités UQAM, https://actualites. uqam.ca

> Asperger's children develop much the same as other children. As they grow, they use different strategies to compensate for the challenges they encounter. This is why professionals who are consulting with them should not be fooled by appearances that might exclude a diagnosis; ask the right questions and carry out a screening that reaches back to early childhood.

Furthermore, I noticed that Antoine seemed more at ease with himself than I had ever felt in similar situations. Indeed, the previous year I had published my first book, and as a result had participated in some literary events. If, on the one hand, I did take great pleasure in the events and being able to discuss writing and the creative process, at the same time I still felt a monstrous anxiety, which weighed upon me terribly. I was so impressed by Antoine's sense of humour and his ability to address the audience, include them and allow them to participate in the event. These were qualities I hadn't thought possible in someone with an autism diagnosis.

After this first contact with the world of this author, I started reading *Musique autiste*. This book contains two distinct, interwoven threads. First, it provides clear information in an accessible format, and second, there is an autobiographical thread in the form of a testimony – two different yet complementary ways of approaching the same subject. The result is an interesting book for adults wanting to find out more about Asperger's syndrome, or who have just received a diagnosis. The book should also be of interest to those close to a person with Asperger's, as well as the professionals surrounding and supporting them.

The second book I read was *The Complete Guide to Asperger's Syndrome* (2008) by the internationally renowned psychologist living in Australia, Professor Tony Attwood, known for his expertise on the subject of Asperger's syndrome. After looking into it, this seemed to me to be the most complete work written on the subject, and therefore the most likely to provide me with a reliable overview. This key work reviews all the characteristics associated with Asperger's. In reading this book I learned that women and girls on the autism spectrum can present differently to boys and men (Attwood 2008, pp.46–48, 53, 74,

81). I would also recommend you do some online research. Several videos of Professor Attwood's presentations and interviews are available, particularly on autistic girls and the internal presentation of autism. Whether in his book or in his verbal communications, he sheds light on the talents and strengths of people with Asperger's, rather than their deficiencies, which is significant. This book is indispensable for anyone who wishes to understand Asperger's syndrome in its entirety.

The third book I became aware of was *Pretending to Be Normal: Living with Asperger's Syndrome (Autism Spectrum Disorder)* by Liane Holliday Willey (1999), a doctor in educational sciences who is also autistic. I was first drawn to this book because of its title. On a day-to-day basis, 'pretending to be normal' seems to sum up the experience of many adults with Asperger's, and especially that of women. My second reason for choosing this book to add to my knowledge of Asperger's syndrome was that it was written by an autistic woman. I was keen to find out about the views and daily life of an autistic woman. The specific features and the developmental journey she describes, relating to autistic women and girls, corresponded to my own to an astonishing degree, which is why I started wanting to learn more about this distinctive presentation.

READING TO INFINITY AND BEYOND

The trio of books I have discussed here formed the foundation on which I was able to build an overview of Asperger's syndrome. Later on, I read more widely, and continue to do so, the scholarship on this subject being vast and ever-growing. I am drawn towards a wide range of texts and works, such as articles written by professionals, scholarly studies, testimonies and, of course, a selection of other books. It is worth noting that I only read a little English before my interest in autism was sparked. Because I am interested in very specific subjects at the heart of this huge assortment, because some scholarly articles are published only in English, and because there were few works in French on the subject when I started reading, this motivated me to work on my ability to read English. It is the same for presentations and conferences that are available online. Improving my English through my interest in this subject came as a bonus that opened the door to an abundance of information and a wide range of documentation.

CHAPTER 10

Key Themes

It isn't possible to say everything or shed light on everything that I'd like to over the course of this piece of writing. In this chapter, I have therefore selected a few points that have stuck out for me – in other words, those with the most pronounced repercussions or that best illustrate some aspects of Asperger's syndrome, and which I'd like to share.

DETAILS, MORE DETAILS AND PUZZLES

Although I love writing, writing a book is arduous for me in the sense of how to put it together. One aspect of my functioning adds to this difficulty.[1] Like many other autistic people, my thinking is detail-oriented. Details dominate my perception and my analysis of objects, facts and situations. This also happens when I am writing. The longer a text I am working on gets, the more challenging I find it to handle and structure. My proximity to and fondness for the detail means I have difficulties when it comes to work on the text as a whole. In a general sense, it is rather like my brain is treating each piece of information, whether perceptive, sensory or other, like a macro photo. So I tend to work on my text as though it is an accumulation of macro photos. Every now and then I have to think to pull myself out of this magnified universe to be able to link up the different sections of the text.

When editing my text, I often come across a passage and have to start reading the whole thing over again to try to make it work on the

---

1   This feature can also become a strength in certain circumstances, including in the case of writing, because being hyperfocused also means being meticulous.

macro scale. I also handle the micro simultaneously, which makes a linear narrative difficult. This is one reason why I prefer to work on short texts – fragments – while devising a structure that can accommodate these texts as a whole.[2] It is a way of working that respects my functioning, which is naturally detail-oriented.

I am using the example of writing to illustrate this characteristic, because I made the discovery while observing the different processes involved in producing my Master's thesis in creative writing. Following on from this discovery, I realized it didn't only relate to the writing process, but it also leaked into every area of my life. The literature course, and the later uncovering of my Asperger's syndrome, increased my awareness and understanding of this way of seeing the world.

I have also noticed that this way of giving precedence to the detail is different from the people around me who have a more typical functioning. For example, if I go for a walk outside or in the woods, a multitude of elements catches my attention: unusually shaped or coloured stones, gnarled roots, textured bark, leaves nibbled by insects, the effects of light through the leaves on a tree, shadows, agitations or reflections on the surface of water, etc. I feel a sort of meditative enthusiasm in observing these things.

In my meditations, I try to see if there is a link between the phenomena I have observed, and I reflect on the way in which these elements fit together. I like to understand how natural systems work. My mind works by means of hypotheses, like building a puzzle until there are enough pieces in place to arrive at a likely or definitive conclusion. This is a natural process for me, and it seems to be quite common among people with Asperger's: 'In cognitive terms, the person can sometimes identify details and notice connections that are not perceived by others who have a different mental framework' (Attwood 2008, p.242).

Over the long term, this process will produce a detailed and sometimes very speedy analysis of a range of situations. It makes me think of detective work that I am carrying out instinctively, regardless of what is under consideration, or the circumstances. In the same context, my partner, who is not autistic, would pay attention to more general aspects of the countryside or footpath. We often discuss this, and he doesn't ask himself the same questions as I ask myself, and doesn't

---

2   Like a constellation, a mosaic or a puzzle.

feel the same need to play the observational, analytical or jigsaw puzzle mental games that occupy my thoughts and fascinate me.

HEIGHTENED SENSES

The topic of details leads me on to another major theme that I have already mentioned, and which has impacted on me my whole life. It is a characteristic that in some circumstances can be a strength, and in others can be felt to be limiting and constraining. I am referring to the fact that my senses can be hugely more sensitive than those of a non-autistic person. A long time ago now, I noticed differences in my senses of sight, touch, hearing and proprioception, but I couldn't clarify my thoughts on them, and I certainly couldn't put it into words. This is something that has an impact on my day-to-day life, and that for a long time wasn't understood by me, the people around me or the professionals I had met along the way.

To introduce this topic, I have decided to quote Liane Holliday Willey, who describes an experience close to my own, even if there are differences:

> I also found many noises and bright lights nearly impossible to bear. High frequencies...clawed my nerves... [S]trobe lights, flickering lights, fluorescent lights; each seemed to sear my eyes. Together, the sharp sounds and the bright lights were more than enough to overload my senses. My head would feel tight, my stomach would churn, and my pulse would run my heart ragged until I found a safety zone. (Willey 1999, p.26)

In my everyday life, I don't know what it means to live with a sensory system that doesn't cause grief. Besides, for a long time I was unaware it was any different for other people. In fact, I had grown up with the notion that most of the people around me managed to cope easily with this intrusive sensory input. For most of my life, I forced myself to mask and put up with it all. That is, until it all became too much. At the age of 29, I grew seriously ill, and afterwards I found I could no longer compensate – in other words, since that episode I couldn't camouflage my traits with as much skill or stamina as I used to, and I can no longer tolerate anything that exceeds my capacity for sensory input. So the problems associated with this hypersensitivity became more prominent, and regularly affected my physical and mental health, consequently limiting my ability to recover. This aspect played a major role in my decision to proceed with seeking a diagnosis.

For some autistic people who, like me, have significant hypersensitivities and who find themselves thrust into a situation that sets off several senses simultaneously, any additional sensory input can become a truly explosive cocktail. The sensory overload experienced by autistic people is still little known or understood. However, it is essential to take this into account, because these experiences have a direct impact on our equilibrium and well-being:

> Many a time autistic individuals have been 'pushed' beyond their limits of sensory endurance. Often this is due to those relating to them not having understood how 'painful' it is to be overloaded by too much sound; visual stimulation; emotional or/and physical demand and environmental expectation. (Lawson, 2003, p.11)[3]

TO FIND OUT MORE

To read an account of what somebody with Asperger's can go through in a situation of sensory overstimulation, see 'Autisme Asperger, un diagnostic à l'âge adulte?' ['Autism, a diagnosis in adulthood?'] by Ann May [Annyck Martin] (2017) on the blog 'Regard9'.

Olga Bogdashina, who has a PhD in sciences and is the mother of an autistic child, goes so far as to put forward the idea that autistic people who repeatedly frequent settings that don't take into account their sensitivities live in an almost post-traumatic atmosphere (2003).

Reading books on Asperger's syndrome, I began to recognize more precisely my sensory specificities as well as how they manifested themselves. Knowing more about these aspects of my functioning has enabled me to communicate them to my loved ones, and others if the situation required it. Previously, I experienced it, or, to put it more precisely, I suffered it, without being able to express what it put me through. My

---

3   Wenn Lawson, psychologist (and autist), in the Foreword to Olga Bogdashina, *Sensory Perceptual Issues in Autism and Asperger Syndrome* (2003). Note that a second edition of this book was published in 2016. Wenn Lawson is a transgender person who signed herself Wendy Lawson at the time, but today goes by the name Wenn Lawson.

own lack of understanding would trigger terrible anxiety, make me feel frustrated and didn't give me any way of adapting or compromising.

Since then, I have refined different strategies that help me manage these aspects better. For example, when I am attending an event that is demanding in terms of social interactions and multiple stimuli, I try to schedule some time for rest beforehand and some time for recuperation in the hours and days that follow. I also try to remain alert to signs that tell me I'm in need of a break, and, instead of pushing myself over my limit, as I had done for so long, I allow myself periods of time to withdraw from proceedings if it becomes necessary. Knowing myself better, I can make better choices of activities, depending on my health, levels of fatigue and levels of anxiety. Overall, since identifying these aspects, I listen to myself more, and I end up respecting myself better.

It can happen that behaviours linked to the sensory specificities of autistic people are poorly understood by the people around them, especially during childhood and adolescence. When this occurs, the behaviours can be attributed to character defects, such as tantrums, rather than as being a difference of neurological function. These offences are liable to cause irritation, jokes and criticism, which, by force of repetition, can damage the autistic child or young person's self-esteem and self-confidence to the point that they come to believe that they aren't a good person, or that they're inadequate or defective in some way. In adulthood, this can translate into associated problems, such as anxiety, depression, social phobias, obsessions and compulsions. This is why it is important to inform those around the autistic person and help them get to know these aspects, so that they can respond appropriately, to reduce and hopefully eliminate unnecessary suffering.

CONNECTIONS, DISCONNECTS AND COMMUNICATION

In therapy, I mentioned to Jonas that I was having difficulty communicating. He seemed surprised at this, and insisted that I expressed myself clearly. At this time I didn't yet have the words to translate how I felt inside or make people understand the problems I encountered – and still encounter – in this area. Since then I've had the time to reflect on it, and this is my verdict. In reality, my ease with communicating varies according to context. In certain situations, I can hold normal conversations, dialogues and discussions on a range of topics. In other situations, such as when I need to share something 'live' from my inner world – in other words, something that requires simultaneous translation – it is more complex for me to communicate. The same thing happens when I have to express myself while tired, sick, stressed or very anxious. In these exact circumstances, my access to my words and the whole of my personal resources is altered, which is to say that it is momentarily reduced or inaccessible.

As a little girl, I spoke very little outside the family circle. My parents described the way I reacted in social situations as 'freezing up'. For instance, when a stranger spoke to me, I would abruptly lower my head and not reply. I remember how that felt on the inside. It was as if my ears had hatches that would close up, as if reality was suddenly put behind a screen. I was there, but at the same time I was elsewhere. Mostly, I stared at the ground, whether at the grain of the wooden floorboards, the patterns on the carpet, or the pebbles on the ground if I happened to be outside. I also took to examining the shoes and trouser hems of the people around me. It felt rather like I was withdrawing and winding up like a coil inside of myself. It caused a sort of cutting off or disconnect on the level of hearing and communication. When I found myself freezing up, it wasn't just that I didn't reply; it was also that I didn't even hear the words of the person who was talking to me to begin with. It was one behaviour among several that took others by surprise and that contributed to my being perceived as a wild child or difficult to approach.

Very few of the adults around me when I was a child were in a position to recognize these behaviours as stemming from a difference in sensory processing or raised anxiety levels rather than simply a refusal to speak or bad manners. With the knowledge we now have on children with Asperger's, I am hopeful that attitudes will change. In this way, young people today, and future generations, will be able to benefit from a greater acceptance of who they are. Guidance, rather than castigation and criticism, is, in my opinion, the way to improve the chance of progress and positive outcomes, as much for the autistic child and their family as for society at large.

I wasn't any more talkative as a teenager, either. On the day-to-day, of course I spoke, but there was at the same time a huge part of me that remained silent. Most of the time, I think I used my silence as a veil or shelter. It gave me a break, some space for peace and quiet, away from the commotion of life. I was a secretive teenager, powerless when faced with the changes to group dynamics that occur around the time of puberty.

> There can be differences in sensory and information processing between autistic people. The sentiments of Jade, age 11, express some of these features well:
>
> > I only use one sense at a time... You need to know that even if I am not looking at you, I am listening closely. That if you ask me to look at you and listen at the same time, I will see you, but I won't be able to hear what you're saying.
>
> The original video clip source of this quotation shows 'the importance of considering the particularities of information processing for autistic people. By reducing stimuli and demands, we can encourage better communication, helping the social integration of each and every one' (Poulin 2015).

This difficulty I have with communicating, even if is not very apparent these days, has been a determining factor in my journey. This problem lay at the root of decisions that have influenced my life course. At the age of 16 I read a book on the subject, which was to have a big influence on my early career decisions. Of the many books I read during adolescence, this one left a particular impression on me. It was *One Child* (Hayden, 1980), written by a special education teacher who told the story of a little girl immured in silence. As I read this book, it moved me profoundly, to such a degree that I started to find out what career paths might correspond with the work this teacher did. This is how I discovered special education as a possible career, and I took steps towards studying in this field.

It was through reading this book that I also found out about the concept of situational mutism (also referred to as selective mutism).[4] Yet there was a strong resemblance between the 'freezes' I experienced as a little girl and what the literature described on the subject of mutism. Years later, while reading on the subject of Asperger's syndrome,

---

4   The term 'selective mutism' is the one used in the DSM-V. However, as it suggests that mutism is a choice, when in reality it is not (the child does not choose not to speak in certain circumstances, it is rather that they cannot), more and more professionals and people are using the term 'situational mutism', which is closer to reality. This video by a specialist in mutism seems to explain the issues around this well: https://www.youtube.com/watch?v=dUorXRBvLlY

I was surprised to discover that many people with Asperger's have experienced this difficulty with communication. Professor Tony Attwood explains the phenomenon well: 'Autistic Children who develop selective mutism in their early years can talk fluently when relaxed, for example at home, but when in school, their level of anxiety is so severe that they are unable (not unwilling) to speak' (Attwood 2008, p.140). He even suggests some pathways for interventions on the subject: 'Treatment programs should focus on which aspects of the context provoke anxiety, and developing strategies to encourage relaxation and confidence' (Attwood 2008, p.140).

According to Professor Attwood, '[g]irls are more commonly affected by selective mutism' (Attwood 2008, p.140). In an episode of mutism, underlying anxiety not only affects speech but can also create a short-circuit in other functions, such as the instant access a person has to multiple nuances and internal resources, a function that will be restored once their feeling of internal security returns. Although I no longer experience 'freezes' in the same way I did as a child, I am still experimenting with what is left of them. They can occur at particular times – for example, when the situation and the challenges in front of me momentarily exceed my capacity for dealing with and responding to them. To go further into this subject, I suggest a video entitled 'Autism and Situational Mutism (when words don't work!)' by Paul Micallef, founder of Autism from the Inside, autistic life coach and aerospace engineer.[5]

In the course of my reading on the female and internalized presentation of autism, I have learned that, like me, many autistic women and girls have a particular interest in reading and writing. Still today, writing is my preferred means of expressing myself alongside a multidisciplinary artistic practice. These are tools and practices I use to ground myself, to centre myself, to get in touch with what's happening inside of me. When the need makes itself known, these devices also help me to get my thoughts in order in such a way that it becomes possible to translate them and communicate them to others. My mode of reflection is based on visual material, such as images or diagrams. This visual thinking allows me to process a lot of information internally very quickly. In my first book, written before I knew that I was autistic,

---

5   See https://www.youtube.com/watch?v=ykIJS-2Vi_Q

I spoke of this type of thinking and communicating in images, which is at work inside of me:

> Firstly, images help me decode and understand what is happening inside me and around me. Secondly, they help me express myself with more detail and accuracy. Images thus act as a go-between: between the chaotic, secret world in which they are born and the conscience (the expressible); between me, my intimate world and the world outside (the others).
>
> By 'images' I mean what I produce in the form of drawings, but I'm also referring to a way of thinking – which constitutes specifically 'thinking and speaking in images'. (Martin 2011, p.31)

Along the way, in reading and finding out about autism, I realized that I'm not the only person to experience this way of thinking. In fact, many people with Asperger's think 'in images'. The author and public speaker Dr Temple Grandin, an expert in animal science, describes her way of thinking as follows:

> I think in pictures. Words are like a second language for me. I translate both spoken and written words into full-color movies, complete with sound, which run like a VCR tape in my head. When somebody speaks to me, his words are instantly translated into pictures. Language-based thinkers often find this phenomenon difficult to understand, but in my job...visual thinking is a tremendous advantage. (Grandin 1995, p.19)

I understood later on that, unlike the majority of people, I have first to translate before I can make others understand how I feel and what I'm experiencing on the inside. This process is not instant, which is why there is sometimes a delay in processing information or any emotions involved, before I can take them into account. Trying to translate my reflections and emotions into words can sometimes cause a sort of crush or log-jam in my thoughts, given that spoken language implies a linear progression, which doesn't suit associative or arborescent thinking as well.

> Arborescent thinking: A way of thinking that deploys several strands of thought simultaneously, generating the proliferation of a network, like the roots of a tree.

I sometimes think of this difficulty in translating my thoughts as an obstacle. Even so, I have built a variety of skills over time, and it's therefore not as difficult to describe my experiences, thoughts and feelings these days as it was when I was younger. Having recourse to written and visual devices unarguably provides support to me. Additionally, writing, and written communication more broadly, has been a part of my life for many years.

It is as a result of this strategy that my social life began to flourish in the second half of my adolescence. I was 15, in 1987, when I had my first live conversation through a computer, one belonging to a technology-mad cousin of mine (communication via computer was still in its infancy at that point). This method of communication immediately entranced me. A few months later I was allowed to install our first modem on the family computer (the good old Commodore 64). The internet didn't yet exist. To be able to connect with another computer, you had to dial up through a modem using the telephone line. You could communicate two different ways using this device: by direct discussion with somebody else with a modem on their computer, or via a bulletin board system (also known as an electronic message board). This was administered largely by teenagers my own age or young adults.[6] At the time, girls weren't often found on this type of network. The platforms functioned much the same way as the forums you still find online today.

This means of communication was a revolution for me. It was much easier for me to communicate in writing than by speaking. Meet-ups were arranged a couple of times a year by the message board users. It is as a result of this new technology that I had my first few experiences of group get-togethers, and that I met my first boyfriend at the age of 17.

This difficulty in communicating was also at the root of other determining choices in my trajectory, notably that of my university studies. Since my primary means of expression is visual, I first got a Bachelor of Arts degree before completing a Master's in Creative Writing. It was during my Master's that I felt at home for the first time in my life. Although writing has since become a cornerstone for me, the visual arts continue to dominate my creative process. In 2020, I started a Doctorate in Art Studies and Practices, with a project that combines several of my interests, including writing and visual arts.

6   Most of them were experts in IT, and it is a safe bet that many will have been diagnosed with Asperger's.

I wish I could have built the strengths I now possess at a younger age. I've been through difficult times and periods of discouragement and latency. It has been difficult for me to make social and professional contributions as much as I would have liked. This difficulty in reaching one's potential is frequently experienced by people with Asperger's, including those who pursue higher studies and who achieve good academic results. The reality encountered further down the line from school, in a professional environment, is totally different. To earn your stripes in the workplace, the required skills extend beyond the scope of what is taught during the Cégep or at university.

> People with Asperger's often have a mixed personality – on the one hand, being very gifted, and experiencing great difficulties or weaknesses, on the other. This disparity tends to cause a lack of understanding among those close to them and healthcare professionals. Some might think that if the person can demonstrate skills in one domain, then it must also be the case in other domains. And yet we live in a society that values qualities and skills based on the social, such as being extroverted and networking, aspects that people with Asperger's find more difficult.

The literary and artistic worlds are no exception to these rules. Talent and hard work alone are not enough to make a place for yourself. These are still very competitive spaces, requiring highly developed social skills. In fact, these days you can no longer be merely an artist or writer. You also have to be an entertainer and salesperson, and know how to network and maintain numerous connections; additionally, you have to be good at admin and marketing. It is a similar story for bursary and grant programmes: they are increasingly allocated to activities on the periphery of creative work, which involves a more developed social awareness, such as running workshops and artistic mediation[7] sessions.

---

7   'In Québec, the expression is used by a growing number of stakeholders to define approaches to building new connections between people and culture. It is an umbrella term for a wide variety of practices ranging from audience-development activities to participatory and community art' (Quintas, E., with Fourcade, M.-B. and Pronovost, M., translated by Roth, K., 2015, p.2).

Quite separately from talent, success in these arenas often goes hand in hand with an ability to build and maintain a significant social network. And it is precisely this skill that many people with Asperger's struggle with. Unless you have the financial means to pay for professional representation,[8] or know an extrovert who is willing to act as an intermediary, or can find colleagues who will be generous with their time and their own networks, it is difficult for adults with Asperger's to integrate themselves fully into creative and intellectual professional spaces. The challenge is all the greater when the person doesn't have a good understanding of their own functioning.

In spite of the obstacles, it is important to stay hopeful and to take actions, at your own pace, to build the life you aspire to, and which is true to you. If you persevere, life can have some wonderful surprises in store.

I recall a challenging time I went through in psychotherapy, caused by difficulties making myself understood.[9] I couldn't express to Jonas what I was experiencing, which I found problematic. I got there in the end by using a composition made up of photos and scraps of text. From that point on, I used a notebook to write down thoughts and diagrams linked with my development. Some time after that, when Jonas asked me to stop using writing to communicate, I felt quite lost. I had been using writing and drawing as a starting point or pivot to unblock my speech and get over any obstacles to communication. When he asked this of me, it was a bit like I had had my speech cut off, as though I had been asked to set aside a significant part of myself. At the time, I didn't see the importance of communicating my feelings, and I didn't know that this could have an influence on the course of things. I thought I didn't have any choice. Hence my psychologist never knew of my reaction to his request, so he never had the chance to explain his decision or make any adjustments.

During the sessions that followed, I stopped bringing along my notebook. However, I continued to use it in between meetings and I now found myself resorting to a trick during our meetings. I used an internal system, a sort of mental gymnastics, whereby I 'saw' in

---

8   An agent or agency representing the autistic writer or artist in order to promote their creative works.

9   Struggling to making oneself understood is one of the four characteristics to emerge from a study intended to identify the features of female autists. For more information, see Mandy and Steward (2016).

my mind's eye what I had written or drawn in the week, and I 'read' whatever I could still remember of it. This trick was tedious, but it helped me to follow, in appearances at least, my psychologist's request to communicate more directly.

Some years later, I attended therapy elsewhere and no longer needed to perform these mental acrobatics. After a few years' break and taking other sorts of actions, I decided to continue with Alice, a psychologist with a humanist approach who uses art therapy. I could have verbal exchanges with her[10] at the same time as using writing, drawing and other artistic techniques to express myself and make progress. My life has taken a new direction since I started adapting my activities and environment to my way of being, and lean into my strengths rather than sidelining them. This way of comprehending the world has the effect of building my confidence. I now perceive and feel myself to be more whole.

A NERVOUS AND EMOTIONAL SYSTEM WITH NO INSTRUCTIONS

My emotions have always seemed to me like an indecipherable magma, a real can of worms. I experienced them happening to me without understanding that they were signs giving me important information. For a long time, I wanted to be rid of this pile of 'stuff' I suffered in silence and that caused me endless discomfort. I didn't have the key to unlock and make use of them. This caused me immense frustration as well as making me feel angry at myself. I hated myself for being 'made that way' – in other words, endowed with a chaotic emotional inner life stripped of any meaning and that I saw as if it were a foreign language. I wished I could 'read' this sort of information as easily as I could learn new academic subjects and ideas. I felt incompetent. It was a bit like a sensitive, fundamental part of myself was walled up, self-sufficient, incapable of contact with the outside world.

Today, after a lot of work on myself, I manage to recognize and express a wider and more diverse range of emotions than I could when I was younger. Artistic outlets have been an indisputable help in developing my voice and my sensibility.

---

10   And in this context, I found I was quite the chatterbox!

OVERWHELM AND EMOTIONAL BREAKDOWNS

Dr Isabelle Hénault, co-author of this book and specialist psychologist, explains that the expression of emotions such as anxiety and rage, for people with Asperger's, can take the form of very intense breakdowns:

> This is what is sometimes called an escalation. This means that if we took a scale or thermometer graded from 0 to 10, very rapidly we will notice changes. The person seems stable, all is well, and then suddenly, what you see is that a small detail, a small thing occurs and straight-away the person is at the top of their thermometer in crisis, in the midst of escalation.
>
> Sometimes, there will be impulsive actions. Sometimes, not. The person can fold in on themselves as if withdrawing from the world, to manage the situation. (MAtv 2015)[11]

This extract describes two sorts of reactions that people with Asperger's are prone to during moments of overload, whether sensory or emotional, or both. These phenomena are termed 'shutdown' and 'meltdown'. Both are a form of emotional breakdown, an internalized crisis and an externalized crisis, respectively.

'Shutdowns' can be described as a withdrawal into oneself, a sort of cutting off, a disconnection in response to an excess of stimuli, or to emotions that reach an unmanageable degree of intensity. It is a silent reaction during which the person seems less responsive, less present; they can no longer hear what is being said around them, and can no longer respond.

As for 'meltdowns', they constitute a 'noisier' reaction than their counterpart. According to autistic people, they can take the form of upset, tears, anger and impulsive actions.

As a child and young person, I mainly experienced shutdowns. Meltdowns were virtually non-existent for me during my youth. However, I started to present reactions with similarities to meltdowns in adulthood. These started to make an appearance after a series of difficult life experiences that occurred in quick succession. This time of great upheaval had a critical impact on my life. To my mind, there is a 'before' and 'after' this series of events. The onset of what I call 'stress

---

11 Dr Isabelle Hénault's reflections, cited from an episode on anxiety from the series *L'Autisme autrement*, devised and hosted by Marie-Josée Cordeau (MAtv 2015).

attacks' dates from this time. These attacks are unpredictable, intrusive and devastating.

For many years, I only had the vaguest of notions of meltdowns, which are, in fact, responses produced by my body, or, more precisely, by my nervous system, in certain contexts. Traditional psychotherapeutic approaches have been largely ineffective for this type of reaction.[12] It is through my own means, by my observations over time, that I came to understand their function. My reading on Asperger's syndrome has also helped.

Over the years I have identified and made a list of my triggers, which helps me to anticipate and allows me to put in place some strategies to prevent them. I have also discovered ways to defuse them. In the last few years my meltdowns have been fewer in number, and less intense. I consequently feel less vulnerable when they do occur.[13] In an article titled 'Je suis une adulte et il m'arrive encore de faire des crises!' ['I am an adult and I still get meltdowns!'], Mélanie Ouimet, an autistic person and promoter of the neurodiversity movement,[14] gives some advice to the loved ones of an autistic person on how to deal with a crisis or meltdown:

> Experiencing an emotional meltdown is very difficult, as much for the autistic person as for the people around them who bear witness to the hurricane unleashed... Mid meltdown, the autistic person is the only person who needs to release the tension. Avoid speaking to them, asking them questions, or touching them. This would only add new information to process, aggravating the meltdown. The meltdown will pass on its own. (Ouimet 2017)

READING SIGNALS

The stress attacks I mentioned had a terrible effect on my health and my functioning for around 15 years. As I learned more about Asperger's syndrome, I became able to notice and define another feature

---

12 The sudden onset of these reactions seemed to catch Jonas, my old psychologist, off guard.

13 For a long time I perceived them to be a disability; today, I take them more as a sign that something isn't right and needs attention or adjustment.

14 'This movement seeks to increase acceptance and recognition of neurological differences, not as mental disorders or disabilities when compared with the norm, but as a natural divergent functioning' (Ouimet, 2018, p.29).

influencing attacks: I had great difficulty connecting with my physical and emotional signals, evaluating them and knowing how to react to them in real time. It was when I heard Dr Hénault speak about this feature that I realized it is common among people with Asperger's:

> One of the main problems encountered by autistic people is learning to identify the signs that an escalation is happening. In clinic, we do a lot of work to teach people with an autism spectrum condition to decode internal signals, whether in terms of their thoughts, psychology, or physiological signals, to help them to avoid, to be truly ahead of the game when it comes to escalation. To help them better understand what's about to happen, and, if possible, if they are verbal, to communicate it to the people around them. (MAtv 2015)

Some years ago, in a process of socio-professional integration, I asked Sophie, the counsellor supporting me, for help with this. This problem was literally disabling me in view of the health problems I was undergoing.[15] At that time, I was having daily hypos and I couldn't spot the clues that indicated the onset of an episode. I only felt the symptoms once the hypoglycaemia was already well established, and once they were already so intense that they stopped me functioning completely. Although it's ever-present, this difficulty reading the signals tends to be compounded when I am away from home and with other people. In the outside world, and in a social situation, there are so many demands and distractions that it becomes hard for me to connect with my own bodily sensations. During my meetings with Sophie, she often reminded me to check in on how I was feeling. At that time I had returned to work, and the repetition of this simple exercise helped me function better.[16]

A few years later, I had an assessment of my sensory profile and it emerged that I have tactile, auditory and visual hypersensitivity, as well as interoceptive hyposensitivity. It is the latter that is involved in the example I give above. To better understand what interoception is, I suggest visiting Kelly Mahler's website.[17] Kelly is an occupational

---

15 At that time I had become more aware of the challenges I encountered in this area and I was therefore in a position to communicate my needs – which I hadn't been previously.

16 With the support of Sophie and the organization that took me on, I created a tailor-made part-time role for myself, after having had several years out of the job market.

17 www.kelly-mahler.com

therapist passionate about interoception who has developed several tools and strategies on this subject.

OTHER SORTS OF DELAY...

Consciously expending effort to 'plug in' to the signs and decode them to be able to use them as a source of information is demanding. Consequently, I often need time to process my emotions. I am talking about untangling them, letting them settle down, then processing them. This leads me on to another feature: I sometimes experience an emotional 'delay', by which I mean having a delayed reaction several hours or days after the situation or event. Antoine Ouellette outlines similar experiences he has had: 'Still today, my emotional reactions are delayed. In the moment of the event, it's possible I won't show a reaction. It is only some hours later that I can get hold of my emotions, and even then, they're only vague and imprecise' (Ouellette 2018, p.53).

Another form of desynchronization I encounter on occasion concerns the divide between what shows on the surface and what is happening on the inside. This feature, which is often inconsequential, has previously caused me some problems. For example, in 1999, when I was 27, my brother died suddenly. In the days immediately afterwards, I told a friend what had happened. After hearing what I had to say, she told me how strong and brave she thought I was being, and that if it were her, she would surely have fallen to pieces. I was speechless at her words, so great was the contradiction with how I felt inside. With hindsight, I realized that I had told her about my brother dying in much the same way as if I had told her I'd gone shopping, bought bananas, cheese, vegetables... Basically, I had told her about it in an automated way, while on an emotional level I was facing up to a colossal wrench.

I had similar difficulties in 2001 when I was undergoing serious health concerns. I tried to describe what I was experiencing as precisely as possible to doctors and friends and relatives, but I did it in technical – even didactic – terms. My method failed to communicate the intensity of the pain and distress I was in. In retrospect, I now think that if I had presented with more typical non-verbal language – in other words, in step with what I was trying to communicate – some medical and psychological issues could have been treated sooner, thereby having fewer repercussions. These days, if I notice that this delay is happening, I am better equipped to mention it, which helps greatly.

ANXIETY AND ITS HEALTH IMPACTS

As far back as I can remember, anxiety has always been part of my life. It has manifested itself and expressed itself in many ways. In one of her books, Temple Grandin articulates that she has the sense of having been born with a nervous system functioning in a constant state of fear and anxiety. Here is what she says on the subject:

> I now realize that because of the autism, my nervous system was in a state of hypervigilance. Any minor disturbance could cause an intense reaction... As I got older, my anxiety attacks got worse, and even minor stresses triggered colitis or panic. By the time I was thirty, these attacks were destroying me and causing serious stress-related health problems. (Grandin 1995, p.111)

Until I turned 40, I was unaware that an underlying factor was intervening in the anxiety I was encountering: an autism spectrum condition.[18] At different moments in my journey, I have had considerable, even incapacitating, health problems. Some of the episodes of ill health have either been triggered by or amplified by unmanageable stress situations. Conversely, the very fact of having had health problems that impacted my daily life and activities over a long period of time has also generated significant anxiety in me.

Grandin testifies to the fact that taking a low-dosage antidepressant changed her life by considerably reducing the severity of the anxiety episodes she experienced. For my part, I haven't seen any conclusive benefits after trialling various medicines. Which brings me on to the point that people with autism and Asperger's can react differently to medicine. My journey is littered with atypical reactions to medication, and for a long time I've been wondering why this is. The result is that I've ended up extremely reluctant when I have to take a new medication for a health concern: 'An atypical response to prescriptions (whether the absence of reaction, or paradoxical effects or hypersensitivity) for psychotropic medications must be considered

---

18 My anxiety triggers differ in a number of ways from those that are problematic to non-autistic people.

a warning sign [of a possible adult autism spectrum condition]' (Le HAS 2011, p.17).

Specialists have also remarked that 'people with autism often require lower doses of antidepressants than nonautistic people... Some only need one fourth to one third of the normal dose' (Grandin 1995, p.119). I noticed something like this while taking certain ordinary medications. I often require a weaker dose than that usually prescribed, or that taken by people I know, to achieve the same effect. Moreover, if I take the usual prescribed dose of the medicine, it will cause me problems, as if the concentration is too high for what my body is capable of absorbing. I would like to understand the physiological processes that can produce these effects. If a doctor or specialist reading this book has any information on this subject, I would be grateful if they could let me know.

EATING DISORDERS AS EMOTIONAL REGULATION

The existence of a past or present eating disorder is widespread among autistic women and girls. The scientific literature states that is a common co-morbidity: 'Some estimates hold that as much as 20 percent of people with enduring eating disorders have autism. Because girls with autism are frequently underdiagnosed, it's often an eating disorder that first brings them to clinical attention' (Arnold 2016).

To summarize, I had two episodes of eating disorders: first between the ages of 17 and 20, and second from 29 to 30. It was a method I had found to cope with immense tensions that were building up inside of me. During my second eating disorder episode, I sent a request for help to a specialized clinic and I was able to receive treatment by following the numerous courses of action they suggested.[19] Since then I haven't had any more episodes like this – in other words, I no longer make myself vomit and nor do I deprive myself voluntarily of food.

However, I still have some rigidities. For example, I often eat the same food or the same types of meals, and at the same times. One factor influencing this habit is health symptoms that I manage in part through diet. In general, I try to prevent pain or other problems I have when I eat certain dishes or foods, just the same as I try to avoid

---

19   Group therapy sessions with psychoeducation, individual cognitive-behavioural therapy sessions, nutritional support, etc., on a weekly basis for a year as an outpatient.

hypoglycaemia.[20] Some traits linked to autism and anxiety probably have an influence on this behaviour, too.

SPECIAL INTERESTS

> Some autistic people have a single field of interest, whereas others have several.

In spring 2015 I attended a conference organized by Dr Hénault on autistic girls and women. In her presentation, Dr Hénault informed us that autistic girls' special interests can be less unusual than those of boys. For example, young girls can often be interested in the same subjects or objects as their non-autistic friends. What distinguishes them is the intensity with which a special interest manifests itself, or their way of playing. At this conference, Dr Hénault also mentioned that a fertile imagination forms part of the criteria characterizing the female profile of autism. Although my inner world has evolved since childhood and adolescence, I still have imaginary worlds inside of me that I make use of if I need to recharge my batteries.

As a child, I had several key special interests. First, books, which I have already mentioned. In fact, I taught myself to read at a young age. At age four and a half, I could read fluently. Learning to read precociously early seems more common among autistic than non-autistic children.

TO FIND OUT MORE

Read the article 'Young autistic children can read before they speak' (Ostrolenk 2017) or the original study in English 'Hyperlexia: Systematic review, neurocognitive modelling, and outcome' by Ostrolenk *et al.* (2017).

After that, I developed a great affinity for visual arts and nature. These

---

20 I have had some serious gastrointestinal problems, and I have multiple food intolerances.

three domains (books, visual arts and nature) are still my favourite fields of interest. As a child, receiving art materials as a present had the same effect on me as going into a library or bookshop – that is, a feverish thrill coursing through my body and mind. I loved reading and making. I also devoted many hours to observing flora, fauna and natural phenomena. From the ages of 11 to 16 I also had an energetic passion for human biology (reading medical encyclopaedias aimed at adults).

As a teenager, I developed an interest in fantasy literature. This interest in imaginary worlds is present in many people with Asperger's: 'During adolescence, some Autistic girls (and sometimes boys) can develop a special interest in fantasy worlds' (Attwood 2008, p.181). It is a special interest that can sometimes lead to a flourishing career in the literary or creative worlds, which is why we must, at all costs, avoid normalizing autistic children, teenagers and adults. Their specific characteristics, once recognized, valued and supported, can help them flourish, both personally and professionally.

Once I became an adult, I developed keen passions in particular contexts. For example, when I was pregnant with my daughter, I had a special interest in pregnancy and, subsequently, in breastfeeding. These fields of interest occupied a significant part of my research for around three years and faded away once these stages were over.

Like many late-diagnosed people, I also became interested in autism, particularly the female and internalized autism presentation and the positive impact of diagnoses for adults. For some people with Asperger's, the knowledge accrued in this area can become quite specialized. It can even happen that, on some points, their knowledge is more up to date than that of generalist healthcare practitioners (GPs, psychologists, psychiatrists and other practitioners). This can give rise to embarrassing or difficult situations for the autistic person. When they try to discuss this subject with professionals, or share information, it can happen that this is taken badly by the professional. However, professionals shouldn't feel threatened by this sort of initiative, which is not meant to question their competence. They should instead welcome information and questions with interest and curiosity, and see it as a sign of confidence and an opportunity to learn from each other.[21] This undertaking is more often aimed at opening dialogue,

21 It is not straightforward to try to communicate your internal functioning to somebody else.

working collaboratively, finding support, as well as envisaging new possibilities for development.

The main interest that has been carrying me over the last few years concerns creation and the processes underlying it. My interest in the creative process first emerged in my 20s, when I was studying visual arts at university. I revived this interest in my 30s, when I was studying literary creation. As part of my course, I had to read some texts by writers describing their creative process. Since being introduced to this sort of text, I have never stopped reading works in which writers describe their creative process, whether in literary essays, writers' notebooks or journals, narratives, poetry or fiction. Similarly, I love to hear artists talking about their artistic process. At the same time, I am interested in the way texts are built – their structure, musicality and voice – and in the relationship between writing and the visual arts.

LITTLE QUIRKS AND HABITS

Let's now turn to quirks and habits. I have always had particular habits. For example, when I was a child, in the evening I would arrange all my cuddly toys around me in my bed in a given order. There were so many cuddly toys that there almost wasn't room for me. The feeling of the toys against my body gave me a sense of security and helped me fall asleep. These days, it's the dirty washing pile in our bedroom that has to 'look nice' – in other words, the garments have to be piled up in such a way that they form a coherent mass, with nothing sticking out. When they aren't, it exhausts me visually and bothers me until such time as the assortment has been put back together as it should be.

Other autistic people also have visual specificities. Valérie Jessica Laporte, author of the blog 'Bleuet atypique' (formerly 'Au royaume d'une Asperger') ['Atypic blueberry' (formerly 'In the Kingdom of an Asperger's Woman')],[22] has shared her penchant for polka-dot and stripey clothes, and for symmetry. This is an aspect that can be seen in some of her artistic photography. On a personal level, when I create, I like something that breaks the symmetry. For instance, I like things that work 'in threes'. When painting or drawing, I often try to incorporate sets of three elements, or multiples of three, in my compositions. When I use adjectives in a text, while it is not a hard-and-fast

---

22   www.bleuetatypique.com

rule, I have a preference for using three. The third element 'breaks' the symmetry and adds a dynamic that I find simultaneously surprising and interesting. I am outlining this difference to clarify that the characteristics and idiosyncrasies of autistic people are not all the same.

What we have in common is that we all have particularities, likes and dislikes, but they are not necessarily the same from one person to the next. There is as much diversity in the tastes and preferences of autistic people as there is among the wider population.

Another point that Jonas brought to my attention during our discussions on autism is that I move my fingers and hands a lot when I am talking. When I am not busy rubbing or interlacing my fingers, I am fidgeting with a pencil or a bracelet, or twisting up my scarf... At home, when we are watching television, I sometimes make small repetitive movements, such as jiggling my foot or picking at the skin surrounding my fingernails. I have noticed that when one of these movements stops, another one comes along to take its place. Another tendency comes to the fore when I am listening to a speaker whose presentation is insufficiently supported by visual content: I start to doodle on a piece of paper.[23] This also happens to me whenever I am on a phone call lasting more than a few minutes. In a face-to-face setting such as a classroom, this quirk of mine has led to misunderstandings. From the outside, it might look like I'm not paying attention, but that's not the case at all. When I doodle, on the contrary, I find myself in a state of deep concentration and receptiveness. Over the years, I have gathered quite a collection of scraps of paper filled with abstract shapes, objects and characters.

INTERACTIONS AND SOCIAL CONVENTIONS

Although it doesn't seem like a big deal at first glance, I have some difficulty adopting attitudes and actions linked to social conventions. Sometimes, the more subtle conventions will pass me by completely.[24] At the same time, some seem pointless to me, or senseless and surplus to requirements. From what I have been able to observe across my life, while social conventions sometimes serve to facilitate contact

---

23 At a conference, during a video presentation or while on a course, for example.
24 They pass me by, in part due to the multiple sensory stimuli to be processed in social contexts. These latter occupy a significant portion of my available energy.

and provide some structure to the way we live together, they can also provide a pretext for psychological or emotional violence, such as thoughtlessness, exclusion or baseless criticism. Because of their way of perceiving and thinking outside the norm, their honesty and the fact that they generally attribute less importance to form than to content, people with neurodivergent functioning such as autistic people are especially prone to finding themselves on the receiving end of this type of violence. This is why it is important to be alert to this, and look for solutions to it collectively and collaboratively.

I have never been a conventional person. Even if at some points I have had to fold and look to 'compress' my personality in an attempt to survive navigating the social world, I have never really been able to conform. On the way home from a celebration one time, my daughter told me how different I am in terms of personality and way of being, compared to others in my generation.

Through my experiences, I have learned the hard way that social conventions occupy a particularly significant place during major life events, such as the birth of a child, a marriage or a death. At those times, there are numerous implicit social codes that greatly increase social pressure. A message that I would like to pass on to the friends, family and other people in contact with autistic people is, during events like this, not to set too much store by conventions. We have all got much to learn, much to question as regards missteps and how we conduct ourselves.

> The double empathy problem (Milton 2012, cited in Mitchell, Cassidy and Sheppard 2019) recognizes that autistic people struggle to 'connect' with other people, but instead of explaining it as a problem residing in the autistic individual, this proposition situates the problem as being on the part of society. This supposes that just as autistic people struggle to understand neurotypical people, neurotypical people also struggle to understand autistic people, perhaps because autistic and neurotypical people have quite different experiences.

In a family, or in an organization (at school or in the workplace, for instance), we must be careful not to blame everything on autism. If the autistic person for their part takes responsibility for being vigilant not to use their condition as an excuse for poor behaviour, or for avoiding a task they are capable of doing, then the people around them must also refrain from using it as an excuse to avoid challenging themselves, or offloading their own problems or worries and passing them on (even unwittingly) to the person with neurodivergent functioning. This also goes for professionals working with autistic people. It is not only those with divergent functioning who need to adapt. We all have much to learn. The differences between us are opportunities for learning, change and growth, as much individually as collectively. Our societies and humanity as a whole would be so much the poorer without the richness these differences provide.

Autistic people sometimes have a different take on friendship to non-autistic people. For instance, some are reluctant to use the phone or catch up with friends. This can lead to the other person thinking the autistic person has lost interest in their friendship. I have two long-term friendships that have lasted because of my friends, not because of me. Even if we don't see each other often, these friendships are very precious to me. Some years before I knew about my autism, these two friends told me that they wondered about it at several points, because I rarely took the initiative to make contact. But they told me that they were reassured because each time they got in touch, I always responded with joy. My lack of reflex to make contact has undoubtedly caused many friendships to fizzle out along the way.

Many of my current friends are neurodivergent, or have had an atypical journey, and they don't take any notice of my quirks. Although there are qualities that I tend to look for in friends, such as authenticity, open-mindedness, humanity, critical thinking and creativity, I am not necessarily looking for someone 'the same' as me. I love discovering new universes: they take me away from my own and help me expand my horizons. I also like being around people with qualities I don't possess, but which complement my own, which surprise me and which I can get along with.

When I was studying for my Master's in Creative Writing, so in my mid-30s, I became aware of certain quirks linked to social interactions. Seminars were a place of lively exchange, which I found creatively and intellectually nourishing. I took part fully in the learning activities. However, I noticed that while I found it easy to participate in discussions in the seminar setting, it was quite different when I found myself with exactly the same group of people in informal contexts. When my fellow students and I met up at a cafe during breaks or lunchtimes, I felt lost. They no longer talked about literature and creativity, but anything and everything, and I really didn't know how to deal with that. These moments of talking were more demanding and more anxiety-inducing than those that took place around the table at seminars. During informal discussions, I tended to partially withdraw, either by observing or by trying to engage just one or two people in particular in conversation.

A change of setting therefore also plays a part in how well autistic people can adapt to or make use of social conventions in the expected way. The split in behaviour between one place and another can sometimes be difficult to understand for someone who is around an autistic person in different circumstances. I know for my part that my ease or unease in one environment or another has sometimes led to questions from the people around me. These days I have a better understanding of the reasons why I can show myself to be active and eloquent in some places and feel paralysed or withdrawn in others.

ORGANIZATION, TRANSITIONS, ROUTINES AND COORDINATION

On a yellowing, lined piece of paper in a photo album from my childhood, my mother has written: '3 years old: generous and messy' beside 'little savage', the family nickname I'd been given. I can remember being a child who was simultaneously well organized in certain things and disorganized in others, a paradox that follows me to this day. I can be very precise and exacting in some activities and at the same time be lax in how organized I am overall.

In the literature on Asperger's syndrome, the information given relates to difficulties with executive function. To put it more precisely, this translates to the following: on the one hand, I can achieve excellent results in very particular intellectual or creative tasks, while, on the other, I struggle to plan my daily tasks, such as washing, housework and organizing my work. A portion of the household tasks is seen to by my partner. It may seem incongruous, but I completed higher studies while having an organizational deficit. Late on, in fact, I developed a working method. But up to that point I just didn't have one.

When I was a teenager, my study method was very simple: I read through my lesson notes the evening before, or even on the morning of an exam. While sitting my exam, I could 'see' in my head the text-book pages and lesson notes I'd taken in class, which enabled me to answer the questions well enough. I got good results, so I couldn't see the point of revising further ahead.

I think that if I had been able to devise a study method more aligned with my natural functioning at an earlier age, it would undoubtedly have helped to balance my life and my leisure and work activities, and would have contributed to my overall well-being. For that to happen, the educational system would have to be rethought in such a way that people with a functioning like my own are motivated to do things differently (by advocating for a pedagogy through self-chosen projects, for instance). As I learned about my functioning late on, I had to keep a constant eye on balancing out my various activities.

This leads me on to the subject of transitions between different activities. I can struggle to 'get into' a particular task or activity, just as once I get involved in it, I have great difficulties 'coming out' of it. When I start writing, for example, I become totally immersed in my project. It starts to live inside of me, to occupy my thoughts permanently, including when I am eating, showering, or even at night.[25] If I could, and if my body and mind let me, I would do nothing but write until my project is completed. But our bodies, minds and lives are just not built like that. To bring my project to fruition, I have to tear myself away from it and take breaks, breathe, move, nourish myself, sleep, complete household tasks, take care of my little family, see friends, etc. But it remains the case that transitions are not easy. Unanticipated interruptions can increase my stress level, especially if they are sudden or occur repeatedly.

In my daily life, I need a particular routine to function well. In a television programme on Asperger's syndrome, one woman explained that she visualized her week by organizing it into little boxes. When she received an invitation or something unexpected came up, she would have to move some boxes around in her timetable, which took her some time to adjust to.

I watched this programme with my daughter, and just before the woman described her system of boxes, I had explained exactly the same phenomenon in my own words. We had a good laugh at the

---

25 I keep a notepad hidden under my bed, ready to jot down my thoughts.

coincidence. It provoked a lengthy discussion with my daughter, and gave her the opportunity to share her experience living with an neuro-divergent mother. In short, my daughter told me that she felt she knew the subject of the programme well, and she shared some stories with me. For example, she told me that when she was younger, unlike how her friends were with their mothers, she would need to forewarn me several days before a friend came over. If a friend phoned her and spontaneously suggested doing something together, it was as if my brain had frozen. I had problems processing the information. These unexpected sudden changes were too fast for my 'little boxes'. I needed to be informed in advance so that I could move my planned activities around and 'remake' a new timetable for the day in my head. Otherwise, anxiety would creep in, and I would no longer be able to think straight. My brain was somehow 'freezing up'. One positive note is that my daughter didn't seem to be unduly affected by this particularity, which she and my husband gently teased me about.

I want to move on to talk about physical activities and motor coordination. As a child and adolescent, I did well at school. However, it was quite a different story when it came to physical education. Sports were my nemesis. If I had been able to skip them, I would gladly have done so. As far back as I can remember, I have always struggled to feel good in my skin and to fully situate my body in the environment in which it finds itself. What I perceive doesn't always match up to my bodily sensations. Some autistic people have difficulties with their fine motor skills. As for me, it's the opposite problem. I developed an aptitude for craft at a very young age, which required meticulousness, precision and dexterity. However, it was quite different for my gross motor skills. While not catastrophically bad, they are nonetheless below the norm.

When I was younger, I did notice certain differences, but I couldn't understand what it meant, and nor could I explain it clearly. Since then, I have found an example that illustrates this difference in motor skills. Around the age of 16, I went on a winter school trip. Once we were up in the mountains, the pupils who had never skied before had to complete a short course before being allowed out on the ski runs. There were about 10 of us who had never skied before. After a while, everyone apart from me had been given permission to go on the main ski runs. What happened here was quite simple. I could conceive in my brain how to position myself to make a snowplough, but I couldn't transpose this idea into physical posture and movement. Despite numerous attempts and my ski instructor's patient direction, I would hurtle down the tiny slope at top speed, totally out of control. The instructor was so worried for me that he accompanied me down my first real descent of a beginners' slope.

My lack of achievement in this sort of activity discouraged me from sports at the time. I would have loved to have got the taste for physical activities from a young age, and found some in keeping with my temperament. Including regular physical activity in my healthy living routine is something I am still working on to this day, but I remain hopeful.

CHAPTER 11

Looking for Answers

AFTER THESE FIRST READINGS

After several months of research and analysis, I came to the conclusion that I didn't present the classic autistic profile, albeit that based on male criteria. Some characteristics matched me, but not all. At the same time, I couldn't eliminate autism as a hypothesis. My investigations continued. I noticed several similarities between the specifics of my development and those described by autistic girls and women. I also recognized some functioning in myself similar to that seen when giftedness is mixed into the picture. At the age of 20, I had, in fact, been admitted to Mensa on the basis of an IQ test, the results of which were in the 99th centile (an average IQ is around the 50th centile).

My investigations were therefore at the meeting point of three precise parameters – in other words, the combination of 'adult', 'female' and 'giftedness'. Jonas let me know that he couldn't take the reflection further, given that he wasn't an autism specialist. After sorting through my reading, I felt the need to go and look for more formal information.

To detect autistic functioning in an adult, you have to be prepared look below the surface. This is because compensation and camouflaging strategies may well have become embedded over time. The DSM-5 recognizes that the screening of girls presents its own set of challenges and may go unrecognized, on page 57 of its 2013 edition. As regards giftedness, specialists like Professor Tony Attwood (2008, pp.40, 53) and Laurent Mottron (interview in Barette 2017) agree that people with an above-average intellectual aptitude can be more difficult to diagnose, given their greater ability to disguise their autistic traits.

SETBACKS AND DELAYS

> Psychiatrists and psychologists don't always have the knowledge or tools to assess autism that doesn't fall into the classic criteria.

Having read in several places that it is preferable to contact a specialist with expertise in autistic adults and women for assessment, I carried out some research to discover what my options were. After a few tries, I identified a specialized group that had a good knowledge of these presentations. I had done my reading, informed myself, discussed it with Jonas my psychologist, weighed up the pros and cons, asked for recommendations for autism associations, and discussed it with my partner. In *The Complete Guide to Asperger's Syndrome* (2008), Professor Attwood suggests asking someone who has known you for a long time to complete the Autism Spectrum Quotient (AQ)[1] test in order to get an objective opinion. My partner had a good laugh reading through the little sentences. His results came out similar to mine.

In short, I had done my homework. All that was missing now was a medical referral to get an appointment through the healthcare system with the professional who had been recommended to me. In spring 2012, I wanted to broach the subject with the psychiatrist I had been consulting with alongside my psychotherapy. And that's when it all became more complicated.

Shortly before I requested a referral to psychiatrist #1, Jonas had had a discussion with them and informed me that the latter was imme-diately ruling out a diagnosis of autism, given that I had good abilities for introspection.[2] I didn't understand this argument, since I had read any number of autobiographies by autistic people giving a nuanced account of their inner life. At the same time, learning that my psychi-atrist didn't seem open to exploring the idea made me apprehensive.

---

1   www.psychology-tools.com/test/autism-spectrum-quotient
2   In the past, my psychiatrist had read my Master's thesis on post-traumatic writing, and told me they were impressed by my analyses. I would have liked for them to show confidence in these same abilities and agree to support my efforts exploring autism.

I worried that I wouldn't make myself understood, as had happened in the past.[3]

When I went to the appointment, my anxiety levels were quite high. Knowing that I struggle to communicate my thoughts when I am feeling very stressed, I'd brought some notes along. As soon as I started reading them, my psychiatrist stopped me. They told me it was pointless to discuss this further, since an autistic person wouldn't have shown any anxiety broaching the subject. And yet at this time I was part of a discussion forum on Asperger's syndrome, and everyone on there who had received a diagnosis had mentioned they'd had raised anxiety when discussing the subject with a healthcare professional. Not to mention the fact that I hadn't seen any document mentioning anxiety as a criterion for exclusion.

The remainder of the appointment was very tense. I found it was impossible for me to share the efforts I'd made, and nor could I get my point of view across. The session left me in an extreme state of stress that lasted for several weeks. I had seen this psychiatrist three or four times a year for about 10 years, and this was the first time I had encountered such difficulties. Up until this appointment, I had had a reasonably good rapport with them.

> A study aimed at identifying the obstacles to diagnosis in adults with Asperger's reveals that a fear of being disbelieved by professionals is the most common and the most feared. The study asked professionals to find ways of fostering a climate of confidence among people with Asperger's, especially while investigating a possible autism diagnosis (Lewis 2017).

Over the three years that followed, we broached the subject a few more times. After a while, they came to realize that I did present with autistic traits, and they told me that if I went for assessment I would very likely obtain a diagnosis. They also added that, in their opinion, assessment was a waste of time; that I would be taking the space from someone who really needed it; that it would be different if I was a child; that

---

3   See my discussion of medical situations that were difficult to explain and to resolve on p.109 and p.110.

there's no medication for autism; and that a diagnostic assessment would be pointless and wouldn't change anything.

After our appointments, I was taking notes and I noticed some contradictions in what they said every now and then. This made me feel uneasy. It didn't seem to be truly a dialogue. Because of my perseverance, in the end Jonas suggested I go to my family doctor to get the medical referral I needed – which I did.[4]

Then I contacted the psychiatrist (psychiatrist #2) attached to the specialist autism assessment clinic that had been recommended to me. They informed me that they couldn't see me, as there was a moratorium at the centre they were working at, and that in those circumstances they only accepted new adult patients if they were referred by a psychiatrist, so my GP's referral wouldn't suffice. They then suggested that I take documentation on female autism to my own psychiatrist, and if that wasn't enough, ask for a second opinion. So I gave my psychiatrist scientific studies and articles by healthcare professionals on the female profile. They wouldn't accept them, and seemed offended when I asked for a second opinion.

In all, over the three years, I was never asked about my childhood or my development, and nor was I asked about the traits I had discussed with Jonas, my psychologist, and my request for referral was turned down. The stress I felt during my final appointment with my psychiatrist was one drop too many. The discussion didn't make sense to me. So I took several months out, to think what to do next.

In spring 2015 I came to the conclusion that pursuing investigations, as I had done over the previous three years, did me more harm than good. I therefore cancelled the appointment I had with my psychiatrist. And I decided to put my trust in myself. A few weeks later, I got in touch with an Asperger's syndrome specialist in private practice in the hope of getting myself assessed.

When I decided to end follow-up with my psychiatrist, I was in a bad place. I had the impression that there was no good option, and that consequently I had to choose the 'least bad' option. In the years that followed, when I saw new ventures and developments happening in my life, I started to see things differently. I understood that by taking this decision – in other words, by following my own analysis and gut feeling – I had actually chosen myself.

---

4   My psychologist didn't have a strong opinion either way on diagnosis.

BEING SEEN, BEING HEARD

Here follows an extract from the letter I wrote to a specialist who saw me a few months after I got in touch:

> I am initiating this process of assessment firstly out of respect for myself. It is the next step in a long journey and follows a variety of processes undertaken in public healthcare settings, which didn't allow me to access a specialist assessment, which would help me find some clarity and certainty concerning mild autism.
>
> My expectations in coming to you are the same as what I have been looking for since the beginning: either to be able to talk to someone with an expertise in adult autism, or in the specificities of the female presentation, or in how autistic functioning manifests when someone is intellectually gifted. My investigations centre on the combination of these particular presentations.
>
> The process is more important than the outcome, for me (whether it leads to an autism diagnosis or not): be it feeling at ease sharing my thoughts and questions; finding an interlocuter who will listen to me, take a closer look at the question, help me work through my thoughts; and, finally, that the explanations offered will align with my own lived experience.
>
> I am also looking at what happens next, notably in terms of jobs, social contacts, and the 'stress attacks' I go through, which constitute a majorly disabling factor in my life, and which psychotherapy has not so far been able to resolve in any significant way.

On 6 August 2015, at the age of 43, and at the end of a process that proved both straightforward and respectful, the autism specialist told me: 'Congratulations, you are autistic!' It was the first time I had ever been congratulated for my differences, for the parts of myself that I had silenced and sealed away a long time ago. I felt relieved, and hopeful that I could make progress in the spheres of my life that needed it.

Because of my past experience, I thought that receiving an autism diagnosis would be disapproved of. So I delayed telling my family doctor. But when I did, about a year and a half later, he told me that there was no shame in it. He had just seen a programme on it, and confessed that it was new to him, since Asperger's syndrome wasn't known of at the time he completed his studies. My diagnosis helped him to understand the persistent anxiety I was experiencing.[5] We had some good talks. My exchanges with him, and with Sophie, the counsellor who supported me while I built a tailor-made job for myself, helped me to welcome my differences, and this reassured me.[6]

As I mentioned earlier, a little over two years after my diagnosis, I made contact with a new therapist. When I met Alice, a psychologist who is not specialized in autism, I felt it was essential for me not to sideline aspects of my personality and my life anymore. From the outset, I shared my story with her, the trials I had encountered along the way, as well as my differences. I gave her information and documentation on the female presentation of autism, which she took the time to go through. My life experience and my differences were all taken into account.

I no longer had the feeling of having to fit into a box, or split myself in two. Each time, the material that I brought along was given consideration. I didn't encounter any problems communicating or making myself understood, as I had done previously. Her multifaceted approach helped me make progress. I felt welcomed in all my many aspects, including my literary and artistic sides. It was a reparative experience.

After the setbacks I had met along the way, I needed to find a place where I could be still, to try new things, reorganize my life and rebuild myself no longer against, but in line with, who I am.

EFFECTS AND CONSEQUENCES

Between starting to write this narrative in spring 2016 and revising it in March 2020, something amazing has happened. In rereading my text and updating it, I was astonished to discover I had made several advancements. In fact, these last few years, my life has taken a turn for the better. I am having successes in my personal and professional lives. I am back in touch with my creative side. I embark on and see through

5   My doctor had known me for 20 years. He has recently retired, and his younger colleague who took over is open-minded on this subject.
6   Sophie has been an important figure in my journey; she adapted herself to my personality and to my particularities. With her support, I was able to bring about practical positive change in my life, professionally, socially and personally. I am profoundly grateful to her.

projects like so many adventures. I do things I had never dreamed of.[7] Most often, I feel joy. I have created a network of collaborators and friends. I am progressively rebuilding my confidence in humans. I am learning to adapt my lifestyle and environment to my functioning rather than permanently over-adapting myself. I'm more assertive.

Little by little, I am rebuilding my confidence and self-esteem. I seize opportunities and accept invitations. I feel fulfilled and I live up to my potential by playing to my strengths. I make more jokes. I meet incredible people. I feel both proud and mindful. I feel pleasure in talking with other people – in small doses. I no longer feel guilty about enjoying solitude. I have fewer stress attacks. Sometimes I feel an inner peace. I have learned what works for me in terms of support. I still meet with challenges, but I am filled with the hope of making new progress. All in all, I am happy with my life, which I feel to be more complete. In sum, I am alive again.

I chose to make my voice heard by writing this book, and through several other courses of action, because a journey like my own – in other words, long and complex – is far from the exception. Right now, many autistic women are completely in the dark about their condition. Some are navigating, with great difficulty, the backwaters of the public health system, which understands little of the specificities of their functioning and is reluctant to give them access to specialist assessment. Yet it is known that diagnosis has a positive impact for the most part. It helps you review yourself, review the path you have been on. It will open up access to tailored support and help you develop your own toolkit. A diagnosis can also be a way of protecting autistic women and girls. Because they struggle to read the intentions of others, some have found themselves in abusive situations. Getting to know your strengths as well as your areas of vulnerability will help you make better choices for yourself and protect yourself from risky situations and the associated consequences.

I have written this narrative somewhat in the style of a speech for the defence. A defence for myself, for the child and teenager that I was, always seeking to flatten out my differences, as well as a defence for the woman that I have become, wishing to live my life fully while being true to these same differences. A defence in favour of all those

---

7   Such as conferences and interviews, and participating in a variety of events and committees.

with a neurodivergent functioning and, in particular, autistic women and girls, and all autistic people with internalized presentation.

Autism, even in a mild form, is the pedestal on which all our life experiences are built. If you can grasp this fact, it will lead to a deeper understanding of yourself, both now and retrospectively. It is a way of providing a safe haven for those parts of yourself that are a little bit unusual and that have often been misunderstood or mistreated in the past.

If you are autistic but don't know that you are, it can be difficult to find a key or instruction manual to understanding yourself. Guided reading will not change who you are, but it will help direct your energies to build an environment that is kind to yourself, and which allows you to move forward by embracing your particularities rather than struggling against them. Identifying my autism has helped me to build where previously there had been only a dead end. I hope that more and more autistic women and girls will be able to gain access, without too many setbacks or delays, to this understanding of themselves.

PART 3

GUIDELINES FOR THE CLINICAL ASSESSMENT AND DIAGNOSIS OF AUTISM IN FEMALE ADOLESCENTS AND ADULTS

TONY ATTWOOD, ISABELLE HÉNAULT, VALENTINA PASIN AND BRUNO WICKER

OVERVIEW

The diagnosis of autism has long been a challenging issue. As there are currently no established biological markers, a 'gold standard' diagnosis is presently a best-estimate clinical judgement based on the behavioural presentation of the individual. However, the variability in autism symptoms and the considerable behavioural overlap with other developmental conditions means that diagnosis is not a straightforward clinical task. The correct appraisal of behaviours associated with autism is an inherently subjective task that relies heavily on clinician experience and skills.

The task of providing an accurate autism diagnosis is complicated further by variability between autistic males and females in the expression of the clinical diagnostic criteria. Moreover, various clinical gender biases have been carried forward since the beginning of the diagnostic criteria for autism, making it difficult for autistic girls and women to be recognized and validated by researchers and clinicians.

In recent years, clinicians have also observed that many autistic children and adults perform both conscious and automatic adaptations to autism that can camouflage (or mask) autistic characteristics in daily life and during a diagnostic assessment. Adaptations such as camouflaging autism were first discovered in the autobiographies of autistic women, but we now know that camouflaging autism is not exclusive to autistic girls and women: it can also occur with autistic boys, men and non-binary autistic people.

The guidelines in this book have been commented on and reviewed by a multinational team of clinicians who, over many decades, have specialized in the diagnostic assessment of autism, and particularly autism in girls and women. The team who developed the guidelines wanted to ensure that they have defined an assessment process that is comprehensive in scope, acceptable to clients, feasible for clinicians to administer, and effective and efficient in delivering an accurate diagnosis. They were developed through extensive consultations with Dr Isabelle Hénault and Professor Tony Attwood and detailed observations of their everyday clinical practices.

The guidelines in this book outline a step-by-step process for conducting an autism assessment for teenage girls and women from the time of referral until the results are shared in a written report. They provide a framework that enables an effective and efficient appraisal of autistic abilities and behaviours. The clinical presentation of autism is complex and varies between individuals. In some, the behavioural features of autism are obvious, and confirming a diagnosis is relatively straightforward. In other individuals, behavioural features can be more subtle and, combined with additional clinical difficulties, make an accurate evaluation of autistic behaviours more difficult. Diagnostic guidelines must describe a flexible process tailored to an individual's behavioural presentation and ensure that a comprehensive assessment is conducted to direct future clinical management.

In order to use these guidelines effectively, as a clinician, you must familiarize yourself with the content and ensure that the requisite professional training is achieved and maintained to deliver these diagnostic assessment services competently. While it was necessary to describe an overarching diagnostic framework that could apply to the full range of individuals who undergo an autism diagnostic assessment, we reiterate the importance of tailoring the process to meet the individual's needs, including considering the individual's broader neurodevelopmental features and environmental context.

DEFINITION OF AUTISM

According to the DSM-5-TR® (APA 2022), autism spectrum disorder (ASD) is characterized by deficits in social interactions, verbal and non-verbal communication and developing and maintaining friendships and relationships, and by repetitive patterns of behaviours, restricted interests and unusual sensory sensitivity. The behavioural features that characterize autism are often present before three years of age, but may first become apparent during the school years or even later in life. The developmental profile and symptoms can vary widely in nature and severity between individuals and the same individual over time, as well as being accompanied by mental and physical health problems.

DIAGNOSTIC ASSESSMENT

To ensure that the diagnostic assessment is accurate and efficient for the full range of autism presentations, the guidelines in this book incorporate a degree of flexibility that enables the process to be tailored to the complexity of the individual's clinical presentation. The guidelines recommend two sequential 'steps' for diagnostic assessment. All individuals undergo a Step One diagnostic assessment, which involves collecting clinical information to determine if an autism diagnosis can be confirmed or ruled out with certainty without further investigations. With some clients, it is possible to have a clear conclusion for the presence or absence of the autistic condition at this stage.

Where an autism diagnosis cannot be confirmed or ruled out with certainty at Step One, it is possible to continue to a Step Two diagnostic assessment. The Step Two diagnostic assessment consists of a semi-structured interview exploring and confirming the female autistic phenotype (Questionnaire for the Diagnostic Assessment of Autism in Females, QDAAF) that allows a more in-depth assessment of the areas where diagnostic uncertainty may exist.

Step One: collection of information

Information collected from various sources can significantly assist the development of a comprehensive clinical picture of an individual.

The first step involves the collection of information on all of (but not limited to) the following topics:

- *Medical and health history:* Information from the antenatal, perinatal, neonatal, past and current period that includes any assessments of hearing, vision, physical and intellectual abilities, and mental health conditions.

- *Family history:* Presence of medical, psychiatric and neurodevelopmental disorders (including ASD) among nuclear or extended family members, as well as relevant social and environmental factors (e.g. family violence, substance abuse, etc.); whether any other family members have been diagnosed as autistic.

- *Developmental history:* How the individual has developed during their lifetime in terms of developmental milestones for communication, social and friendship abilities, gross/fine motor and personal care skills, as well as the presence of any developmental regression.

- *Autism-specific symptoms:* Behaviours relating to social communication/interaction and restricted, repetitive behaviour patterns outlined in the DSM-5-TR® or the *International Classification of Diseases, Eleventh Revision* (ICD-11) (WHO 2019/2021) diagnostic criteria.

- *Other relevant behaviours and symptoms:* Information collected from various sources can also greatly assist the development of a comprehensive clinical picture of an individual. These include:

  - Screening to determine if further investigations are required to explore if differential or dual diagnosis should be considered, such as ADHD, anxiety eating, specific learning disorders or depression

  - File review of existing assessment reports, early intervention/medical/psychological reports, parent records of early development (e.g. baby books, home video footage), school records and evidence of any childhood challenges or traumatic experiences

  - Communication with a caregiver or a support person who knows the individual well

  - Medical evaluation of the individual, consisting of

neurological and physical history and examination to assess whether there are medical causes and associations with the individual's behavioural presentation, such as chronic fatigue syndrome, fibromyalgia, Ehlers-Danlos syndrome or catatonia.

Questionnaires and tests

Several screening tests or questionnaires are completed with the client (and with the parents in the case of an adolescent or a young adult) during the clinical interview to ensure a greater breadth of information.

Other psychological and neuropsychological tests and questionnaires, different from the list below, that evaluate specific domains or characteristics of autism spectrum conditions can exist in different countries. They can be added to create a more complete and comprehensive battery of assessments. It is important to choose the questionnaire or test by considering the age, language skills and cognitive abilities of the client.

SCREENING/PRE-DIAGNOSTIC TESTS

The following tests are suggested, but a selection can be made according to your professional judgement. For the complete bibliography of all tests mentioned in this section, see the References at the end of the book.

For children and adolescents (aged 5–15):

- Autism Spectrum Quotient: Children's Version (AQ-Child) (Auyeung *et al.* 2008)

- Autism Spectrum Quotient (AQ) – Adolescent version (Baron-Cohen *et al.* 2006)

- Children's Empathy Quotient (EQ) and Systematizing Quotient (SQ) (55 items) (Auyeung *et al.* 2009; see also Lawrence *et al.* 2004)

- Adolescents' Empathy Quotient (EQ) (Auyeung *et al.* 2012; see also Lawrence *et al.* 2004)

- Adolescents' Systematizing Quotient (SQ) (Auyeung *et al.* 2012)

- Face Test (Baron-Cohen 2017)

- Reading the Mind in the Eyes Test (Baron-Cohen *et al.* 2001a; see also Baron-Cohen, Wheelwright and Jolliffe 1997)

- Faux pas test for children (Baron-Cohen *et al.* 1999)

- Theory of mind test (Happé 1994).

For young adults and adults (16+):

- Autism Spectrum Quotient (AQ) (Baron-Cohen *et al.* 2001a; Stone, Baron-Cohen and Knight 1998; Woodbury Smith *et al.* 2005)

- Empathy Quotient (EQ) for Adults (Baron-Cohen and Wheelwright 2004)

- Friendship Questionnaire (FQ) (Baron-Cohen and Wheelwright 2003)

- Systemizing Quotient–Revised (SQ–R) for Adults (Wheelwright *et al.* 2006; see also Baron-Cohen *et al.* 2003; Goldenfeld, Baron-Cohen and Wheelwright 2005)

- Sensory Perception Quotient (SPQ) (Tavassoli, Hoekstra and Baron-Cohen 2014)

- Face Test (Baron-Cohen 2017)

- Reading the Mind in the Eyes Test (Baron-Cohen *et al.* 2001a; see also Baron-Cohen, Wheelwright and Jolliffe 1997)
  With this test, considering the raw score is not always sufficient; the clinician should ask the client if they gave their answer intuitively or by taking time to determine the most probable answer cognitively (Stone, Baron-Cohen and Knight 1998)

- Camouflaging Autistic Traits Questionnaire (CAT-Q) (Hull *et al.* 2019)

- Social Stories Questionnaire (Baron-Cohen 2004).

Diagnostic assessment tool
For autistic young adults and older adults (18 years old or older):

- Ritvo Autism Asperger's Diagnostic Scale-Revised (RAADS-R) (Ritvo *et al.* 2011)

  This is currently the only diagnostic test that is available for this age range.

AN OPINION ON THE ADI-R AND ADOS

Neither the Autism Diagnostic Interview-Revised (ADI®-R) nor the Autism Diagnostic Observation Schedule, Second Edition (ADOS®-2) have been adequately adapted for our evolving understanding of autism as expressed by many autistic girls and women, and how to recognize the expressions and adaptations, such as masking/camouflaging, that have emerged in the last 20 or more years. Thus, these instruments have been found to miss the more subtle presentations of autism. Results of recent scientific publications show that the ADOS®–2 has low diagnostic accuracy for females, older individuals and individuals with personality disorders or high intellectual ability (Langmann *et al.* 2017).

Thus, ADOS®-2 and ADI®-R are not suggested as the primary or exclusive instruments for a diagnostic assessment of level 1 autism in females.

Supplementary tests for women and girls:

- Questionnaire for Girls with Asperger Syndrome (QGAS) (aged 5–12 and 13–18) (Attwood and Garnett 2013)

- Questionnaire for Autism Spectrum Conditions (Q-ASC) (Ormond *et al.* 2017)

- Autism Spectrum Screening Questionnaire-Revised Extended Version (ASSQ-REV) (Kopp and Gillberg 2011)

- Girls Questionnaire for Autism Spectrum Condition (GQ-ASC) Scale for Adult Women (Brown et al. 2020).

Personal notes: helping your clients write about themselves and their experiences

The client is asked to produce a several-page document describing their current and previous interests, sensory sensitivity, past and present friendship and relationship network, emotion perception and regulation and any challenging aspects of daily life such as coping with change.

The document could include specific questions such as:

- How well do you understand other people, especially regarding their conversational and emotional needs?

- Did you enjoy going to parties/sleepovers/play dates?

- How did you/do you get on with other people?

- How did you/do you get on at school with learning and social-izing?

- Were you bullied, teased, rejected or humiliated at school?

- What things annoyed you as a child/adolescent?

- Was it easy for you to verbally share how you felt about things with your parents or caregivers?

- Did you prefer to play with others or alone or both?

- What were your parents' or caregivers' greatest worries for you as a child/adolescent?

- How good are you at reading social cues?

- Do other people describe you as unaffectionate?

- Are you oversensitive to how someone is feeling?

- Do you prefer to work on your own?

- How do you regulate your emotions?

- Do you have social rules that only you seem to adhere to?

- Do you need a lot of downtime alone?

- Have you often been deceived by others?

The answers to these questions are explored in greater depth during the diagnostic assessment.

Notes from a family member or friend

Family members or friends can be asked to write a description of the client's salient autistic characteristics, some memories of the client's childhood, especially in social situations, and some salient anecdotes of their past/present life.

If the client is an adult who is in a long-term relationship, you may ask the client's partner to complete the screening questionnaires to provide a second opinion. There can be considerable differences between each partner's perception of autistic characteristics as described in these screening instruments. If the partner who shows signs of autism disagrees with the suggestion that they are autistic, they may deliberately minimize their self-rating of autistic characteristics. If the non-autistic partner is convinced their partner is autistic and this provides a potential explanation for their relationship issues that they have been seeking, they may magnify their partner's autistic characteristics.

Medical records

When possible, record a description of:

- Previous medical/psychological diagnoses

- Past and present medications.

A common occurrence in autism is the presence of one or more previous medical/psychological diagnoses, especially in autistic females. Many may have been diagnosed in the past with:

- Depression, especially postnatal depression

- Borderline personality disorder

- Bipolar disorder

- ADHD

- OCD

- Anorexia or eating disorders

- Anxiety and panic attacks

- Social phobia

- Avoidant personality

- Tourette syndrome

- Burnout.

Unfortunately, it is very common for autistic females to have a history of struggles and difficulties that have not been fully and deeply understood and appreciated by health professionals, primarily because of the stereotypes and prejudices connected with autism spectrum disorders and the lack of knowledge about adaptations to autism by autistic girls and women.

When the client presents with one or more of these diagnoses and claims they have never felt entirely represented by any of them, it is valuable information to consider during the diagnostic assessment, as autism may be the missing piece of the diagnostic puzzle.

Conclusion of Step One

Taking into account all information collected, Step One will result in one of the following outcomes:

- There is enough information that the individual would meet the diagnostic criteria for ASD.

- The autism diagnosis cannot be confirmed or ruled out with certainty, and you need to deepen the assessment with specific questions that cover the typically female autistic characteristics in greater depth. In this case, the diagnostic assessment continues with the use of the Questionnaire for the Diagnostic Assessment of Autism in Females (QDAAF).

In some cases, it can also be possible that at the end of Step One, the individual clearly does not meet the criteria for ASD (e.g. when most of screening test results do not meet the cut-off scores indicative of autism and the self-description and family member or friend's description are inconsistent with the autistic profile). In that case, it can be recommended to proceed with a differential diagnosis (personality disorder, OCD, etc.).

Step Two: a specific questionnaire for females

During this clinical interview, information is obtained by asking semi-structured, open-ended questions. As some aspects of the autistic female profile can be missed, underestimated or inconspicuous, most of the themes previously investigated with the tests/questionnaires and the personal notes are reviewed and explored further during this step.

Eight specific topics (Self-recognition as autistic; Childhood and school years; Social interactions; Cognitive aspects; Relationships; Animals; Sensory aspects and perception; Health) will be examined, as described below. All questions for each topic should be asked to achieve a comprehensive clinical portrait. The question sequence is flexible and should follow the spontaneous course of the conversation. However, the 'A' topic (Self-recognition as autistic) should be addressed first.

Two different versions of the Questionnaire for the Diagnostic Assessment of Autism in Females (QDAAF) are presented in the Appendices of this book:

- Protocol 1 is the list of questions divided into eight topics that the clinician will spontaneously use during the clinical interview. The questions can be addressed to the client following a natural conversation and asked in any order.

- Protocol 2 is the list of questions divided into eight topics, with the necessary space to write down each answer that the client gave. This version is used if you, as the clinician, want to follow a specific order of questions.

Below is a description of the typical answers for the 61 questions (plus an additional 10 questions for complementary information about physical health and sexuality) of the Questionnaire for the Diagnostic Assessment of Autism in Females (QDAAF), divided into eight specific topics. The expected answers reflect a common or typical profile of autistic females.

Items of the QDAAF with typical autistic responses
A. Self-recognition as autistic
1. *When was the first time you learned about autism?*

The answers to this question can be very different from one person to another. Some may have:

- read articles or watched television programmes about autism and found some commonality in certain aspects of themselves

- watched YouTube (or other social media) interviews of autistic adult advocates who tell their life stories and describe their daily experiences

- an autistic relative and have started to realize they share similar characteristics

- discussed autism with an autistic student at school or work colleague and began to search for information to better understand their developmental history and profile of abilities, or

- used screening tests on the internet,[1] to confirm autistic traits.

2. *Do you recognize yourself in some aspects of what you have heard/read about autism? If yes, describe in what way.*

It is interesting to know which aspects of autism the client recognizes in themselves. Typically, we have found that autistic women will recognize and describe the characteristics that they identify with, with more self-awareness and openness than autistic men.

3. *Did you ever think you were different from children your age? If yes, when did you start having these thoughts, and how did you perceive yourself as different?*

The typical autistic answer is YES. Autistic children usually start to feel different from their peers when interacting socially and when friendships are expected to become a central part of their daily life (around 6–10 years old). At that stage, their difficulty/inability to make friends becomes more evident. It is common to receive the answer 'I've always been different from other children my age'. Some autistic individuals, especially women, can report a perception of difference from others even before the age of six.

B. Childhood and school years

1. *What memories do you have about your primary school and secondary school years?*

It's important to collect personal information starting from primary school because the difficulties and differences in behaviours and abilities often emerge during this time period. It is possible that autistic

---

1   www.autismresearchcenter.com

women perform well at school in mathematics, science and biology – as these subjects are logical and structured – but we have also recognized that autistic girls and women can be talented in speaking foreign languages and in the arts including fine art, music, writing fiction, dancing and drama. A coping mechanism for autism is to create imaginary worlds (and sometimes friends) and pass hours fantasizing and using the arts to explore and express thoughts and feelings. An autistic woman may have developed her artistic abilities into an established and successful career.

Typically, during secondary school, the differences between an autistic adolescent girl and the other girls become more and more evident and episodes of bullying and teasing are unfortunately a frequent experience.

2. *What memories do you have about being a student at college and/or university?*

The experiences here can be very different to non-autistic students. Autistic women often continue to experience episodes of teasing and bullying. They may focus all their energy and time on their field(s) of study, finding self-identity by what they achieve academically rather than socially.

3. *Was it difficult to make friends? And now?*

The typical autistic answer is YES. Making new friends or maintaining close relationships was and is still a challenge. However, the specific aspect of the feminine profile is the presence of one or two close friend(s) that usually accompany the client's life since she was a child/adolescent. The friendship may continue for decades.

4. *How many friends did you have? And now?*

Friendships for autistic females are usually limited to one or two people, and it is not unusual to find autistic women for whom the only reference person is a partner.

It could be interesting to ask about the frequency of meeting friends, which is usually less frequent than that of neurotypical people, perhaps only once or twice a year. Many autistic people have only online friends and prefer this type of friendship, which avoids face-to-face interaction.

5. *Did you have an imaginary friend? And have one now?*

Autistic women who had an imaginary friend in childhood may continue to have imaginary friends in their adult years. The role and function of this friend were/are to guide her actions, to be an individual other than herself to whom she can refer all the times she has doubt about how to behave in certain situations, and to be consulted as needed. Her ideal friend. It is not an expression of psychosis. This vivid imagination and internalization of friendship also serves as a way to 'recharge energy' and to escape from day-to-day difficulties.

6. *Have you ever been the victim of bullying and teasing?*

As described before, autistic women have often experienced episodes of bullying and teasing during their childhood and/or adolescence. These episodes have a deep impact on the subsequent development of their social abilities and confidence. Masking/camouflaging autism can be a way of being part of a social group and thus less likely to be bullied. Bullying also affects self-esteem and confidence and can contribute to clinical depression.

7. *Did you observe other children rather than talk and interact with them?*

The typical autistic answer is YES. A specific trait of the female profile is the feeling of isolation experienced in childhood, which is qualitatively different from avoiding social behaviours usually associated with autistic male traits.

A characteristic of autism is the ability to seek patterns and systems. This ability can be applied to social situations, such as observing and analysing the social behaviour of peers to learn social rules and conventions, avoid making a social mistake and achieve inclusion and friendship. The ability to observe and analyse peers can lead to a successful career as a psychologist.

8. *Did you like to watch films, soap operas or television series to observe and study the characters' social behaviour and interactions?*

The typical autistic answer is YES. Autistic women may learn about social behaviour by observing their peers and avidly watching television and films to study the interactions between the characters. Another way of learning social behaviour is to read fiction describing the character's thoughts and feelings and social conventions and expectations in the text. Autistic girls and women may have always enjoyed reading fiction which is an indirect way of exploring social interactions without the risk of making a social mistake as can occur in real life.

9. *Did you have one or more people/characters that you used as models of behaviours?*

The typical autistic answer is YES. It is not unusual that, after asking this question, the client explains how she has always mimicked a person (that could be the mother, the older sister, a teacher, etc.) or a character (from a film, a book or a television series) that she considered as a model of good social behaviours to imitate.

10. *Were you a child who preferred to be alone and being in your imaginary world?*

The typical autistic answer is YES. Most autistic adolescents and women spend hours and hours imagining, replaying and rehearsing social interactions in their mind, based on what they have seen or learned. If it's so difficult to understand the social rules of the real world, to be appreciated and valued, why not escape into your imaginary world? This characteristic can remain and develop over time, and become a central part of their lives. This may lead to a career as an author of fiction.

11. *Did you try to interact with girls of your age and become friends but frequently without success?*

The typical autistic answer is YES. Some autistic women remember having tried a lot of times to interact with the other girls and to make friends but with little or no success. They were seen as odd or 'different', and peers were often uninterested in becoming their friends. They were not 'cool'. For many autistic women, the only relationships they had during childhood were with adults or pets.

12. *Did you experience episodes of situational mutism as a child or adolescent? And now?*

It is not unusual to find autistic women who experienced a period of situational mutism as a child and even as an adult. This involuntary mutism can be a symptom of extreme social anxiety with the response of 'freeze'. Some autistic women can still show episodes of situational mutism, especially in association with social events where they are confused and overwhelmed.

13. *Have you ever been interested in boys (or any other kind of romantic relationships)? If yes, when did you start?*

Some autistic female teenagers have been described as 'tomboys', preferring the company of boys whose social rules are relatively simpler than those of girls and having a 'tomboy' look or attitude. Unfortunately, this can lead to a misinterpretation of their social/sexual preferences and desires by their peers.

Not all autistic women show an interest in romantic relationships, but when it happens, it is usually a late interest (around their 20s–30s).

In some cases, they have had aversive sexual experiences due to social immaturity and the inability to identify the intentions and actions of others and recognize and state their sexual boundaries.

Another important aspect to consider is the possibility that some autistic women use their sexuality to attract attention or relationships. They can learn that their sexuality can be a way to obtain a connection and engagement with other people. Hypersexuality can also occur when an autistic adolescent girl or women has difficulties recognizing sexual boundaries or when exploring sexuality by mere curiosity.

14. *What kind of hobbies did you have when you were a child? And now?*

This is a question to find out about her interests or passions. These can function as a source of enjoyment, achievement and relaxation, and act as a thought blocker for anxious or negative thoughts, and provide opportunities for socializing with others who share the same interests.

C. Social interactions

1. *Is it difficult for you to participate in activities with many people (group activities, meetings, events, hanging out with a large group of friends or colleagues, etc.)?*

The typical autistic answer is YES. This is a characteristic of many autistic people. However, while autistic women are often able to successfully participate in family reunions or work meetings, after the event they feel mentally exhausted from masking their autism and using their intellect rather than intuition to engage socially.

2. *Do you feel exhausted mentally and physically after a day/some hours just surrounded by many people?*

The typical autistic answer is YES. This question is asked to determine the mental 'cost' of being in close proximity to other people. Being in a crowded place is a major source of mental energy depletion. However, for an autistic person, two is company and three is a crowd.

3. *After a day/some hours surrounded by many people, do you feel the need to be alone and do your favourite activity?*

Autistic men and women often report that solitude is their preferred way to recharge mental energy.

4. *Do you experience some difficulties following a conversation with two or more people?*

The typical autistic answer is YES. There can be difficulty processing the conversation when people talk over each other. This is a characteristic of autism and is not specific to autistic women.

5. *Is it difficult for you to understand the emotional reactions of others?*

The typical autistic answer is YES. This is due to difficulty reading and processing non-verbal information and social context to determine what someone is thinking or feeling (theory of mind abilities) and predict how they will respond. This autistic characteristic is not gender specific.

However, many autistic girls and women have learned to read non-verbal communication by studying books or television series about non-verbal language. Thus, they can perform well in tests of these abilities, such as the Reading the Mind in the Eyes Test (Baron-Cohen *et al.* 2001a) What distinguishes autistic performance from neurotypical is the high degree of reasoning and length of processing time to complete these kind of tasks.

6. *Do people close to you (family, friends, partner, etc.) sometimes tell you that you have too intense of a reaction to a particular situation?*

The typical autistic answer is YES. This is due to difficulty in moderating the intensity of emotional reactions and identifying a more moderate reaction that would be anticipated by others. They may have had to learn effective emotional regulation cognitively.

7. *Is it very difficult for you to have a superficial conversation (social chit-chat) or to talk about general topics (the weather, politics, sport, gossip, etc.)?*

The typical autistic answer is YES. For many autistic people, such conversations are considered boring, inconsequential and a waste of time. It is extremely difficult for autistic people to talk about superficial or general topics. As this is often the starting point of a conversation with an unknown or not very well-known person, it explains one of the reasons why autistic people experience difficulties in initiating conversations and friendships.

Many autistic women have learned how to initiate and maintain superficial conversations, but they will continue to represent a great drain of social energy.

8. *Do you feel like you are practising the social rules and conventions in an unnatural, not spontaneous, way?*

The typical autistic answer is YES. Autistic women, in particular, may have learned to 'act' in social situations as if they were playing a role, with a learned script. This is the basis of the concept of masking or camouflaging, and over time, it leads to clinically significant difficulties in defining their true identity and authentic self.

9. *Is it a problem for you to understand when and/or how to stop a conversation?*

For many autistic people, it is difficult to recognize the social rules that initiate, maintain and end a conversation. Others may report they abruptly end a conversation or do not read the signals that their conversation partner wants to end the conversation.

10. *Do you find it difficult to talk by phone when you cannot see the other person and their reactions?*

This is a typical characteristic of many autistic people. A phone conversation is often perceived as demanding intellectual energy to process unclear or ambiguous information solely conveyed by speech. Autistic individuals often find it easier with the additional information from facial expressions and gestures.

11. *Is it difficult for you to take notes during a conversation on the phone?*

The typical autistic answer is YES, since the double task of listening and writing adds complexity to the conversation due to difficulty multi-tracking, which is an executive function skill associated with autism.

D. Cognitive aspects

1. *Do you think in pictures? Are you a visual thinker?*

The typical autistic answer is YES. Autistic people often report being able to think in images or 'movies' as opposed to verbal or conversational thinking.

2. *Do you tend to see patterns and notice systems more than other people?*

The typical autistic answer is YES. A characteristic of autism is to notice and perhaps be distracted/absorbed by details. This is due to an ability to focus on details rather than the big picture and be fascinated with identifying patterns, which can lead to talent in medicine, mathematics, drawing in photographic realism, identifying errors, and many other aspects of careers that benefit from this ability.

3. *Do you have exceptional long-term memory with details or information that attracts your attention (or connected to your special interest)?*

Many autistic adults will report the ability to store and recall information in their long-term memory (like a hard disk on a computer). On the other hand, short-term memory abilities (working memory and especially auditory memory) are often more limited. A quality of autism is having expert knowledge that can contribute to a successful career where specialist knowledge is valued.

4. *For you, is everything 'black or white'?*

The typical autistic answer is YES. Autistic men and women tend to express this 'all or nothing' characteristic in various fields: emotions (extremes of emotions), relationships (best friend or no relationships), opinions and ideas (there is no 'grey zone').

It should be noted that some autistic individuals will not understand this question because of the use of an absolute term ('Nothing can be ALWAYS the same, so why are you asking if EVERYTHING is "black or white"?') and/or because of the use of a metaphor using the term 'black and white' in a literal way. A tendency to make a literal interpretation is one of the signature characteristics of autism.

5. *Are you a perfectionist? Are you able to find errors where other people can't?*

The typical autistic answer is YES. This is a typical characteristic of many autistic people. This can affect social situations in that the autistic person is notorious for pointing out and correcting another person's error. This can include pointing out the errors of the person conducting the diagnostic assessment. The ability to spot errors can be valued in some careers, such as beta testing of computer programs, accountancy or crime investigation.

6. *Do you feel the need to live and work in an organized and structured environment? Do you feel anxious if your order is changed by someone?*

The typical autistic answer is YES. This is a characteristic of many autistic people and is associated with one of the diagnostic criteria (B2) in the DSM-5-TR®.

7. *Do you have set routines in your daily life? What happens if something or someone changes your routine?*

The typical autistic answer is YES. If the routine changes, the autistic person usually feels unsettled with an increase of anxiety and an urge to re-establish the anticipated order. An autistic person often seeks predictability and can have an intolerance of change and uncertainty.

8. *Are you an honest but also naive person?*

This is a characteristic of many autistic people. The honesty can be a problem in terms of not understanding the value in a friendship or relationship of the concept of a 'white lie'. The autistic person can be notorious for being blunt and direct and not understanding why someone would be offended by knowing the truth. The naivety can be a concern in autistic women having been vulnerable to financial, emotional and sexual exploitation and abuse.

9. *Is it difficult for you to read between the lines in a conversation?*

The typical autistic answer is YES. This is due to difficulty with implied meaning. For many autistic women, since languages and grammar are a frequent special interest, the difficulty is not in understanding metaphors or idioms or ways or speaking, but rather more complex implied meaning like lies, manipulation, exploitation and other social dynamics like flirting or mobbing.

10. *Do you understand what people say in a literal way?*

The typical autistic answer is YES. This is due to aspects of theory of mind abilities – that is, perceiving and processing non-verbal communication and context that provides information on someone's hidden intentions. There can be further discussion of examples of difficulties with idioms, figures of speech and sarcasm.

11. *Is it very difficult for you to tell lies?*

The typical autistic answer is YES. There may be a greater allegiance to the truth than people's feelings and confusion about why non-autistic people lie so frequently.

12. *Do you feel your mind is full of feelings, thoughts or images? Is it difficult for you to translate them into words?*

The typical autistic answer is YES. The term alexithymia describes a characteristic associated with but not exclusive to autism, namely an impaired ability to identify and describe thoughts and feelings in speech. The prevalence of alexithymia in autistic adults is around 50 per cent, while the prevalence in the general population is 5 per cent. Alexithymia is associated with difficulty focusing on and accurately appraising and describing in speech the subtleties and textures of internal emotional states. As an autistic adult said, 'I'm not good at wording my feelings'.

13. *Do you feel like your mind is always working, even during the night?*

The typical autistic answer is YES, and racing and anxious thoughts are associated with sleeping problems, especially delay in falling asleep.

14. *Is it difficult for you to remember spoken instructions?*

The typical autistic answer is YES. This characteristic may lead to difficulties in the workplace or at school and is associated with short-term rather than long-term memory.

15. *Do you like to deeply understand what you are interested in, to precisely understand how things work, to always learn new things and explore them till the moment you feel you have totally understood them?*

The typical autistic answer is YES. When an autistic person finds a topic or an activity that captures their interest, they can spend considerable time deepening their knowledge and becoming an expert in their area of interest.

Each passion will have a 'use by date', which may be hours, days, months or years, and when eventually discarded, will be replaced by another passion.

E. Relationships

1. *Do you use different masks or characters in various situations in your everyday life?*

The typical autistic answer is YES. A non-autistic woman may act as 'wife and mother' at home, as a 'professional' with her line manager and colleagues, and as a 'friendly and fun person' with a group of friends or relatives. However, this natural characteristic of different roles can be taken much further by an autistic teenage girl or woman. They may have developed an interest in observing other females (or people in general) since childhood because they appear as potential behavioural models to achieve social acceptance. They can develop different roles or masks to be used in different contexts or with different people. They become a 'chameleon' camouflaging or 'masking' their autistic behaviours. It can be considered adaptive because it's a natural strategy to navigate daily life, but many autistic women arrive at the point where they feel unable to disclose their autism and be their authentic selves. Moreover, this can frequently lead to autistic burnout or depression. It is at this point that they may consider a formal diagnostic assessment for autism.

2. *Do people close to you (family, friends, partner, etc.) say that you are too direct and without filters, but according to your perspective, you are just telling the truth?*

The typical autistic answer is YES. This characteristic is linked to theory of mind abilities. An autistic person will typically show difficulties in the subtle comprehension of conversation's rules, becoming perceived as too blunt or even rude and impolite. This characteristic does not differ by gender. However, in some cultures, girls and women who are direct, blunt, not submissive or deferential are more likely to be criticized and rejected by their culture for not expressing the cultural expectations of being female.

3. *In your general experiences, are you attracted to people with a strong personality?*

The typical autistic answer is YES. People with a strong or dominating personality are seen as a guide to navigate the social world, determining what the autistic person should do or say. There is no indecision or confusion, only clear direction.

4. *In your relationships, are you attracted to a person rather than his/her/their gender?*

There is a changing conception of autistic gender identity and sexual preferences and attraction. Autistic people, both men and women, may describe themselves as 'gender neutral' and/or attracted to personality characteristics, abilities and interests without complying with conventional expectations of choosing a relationship with someone of the opposite gender and within a specified age range and cultural similarities.

F. Animals
1. *Do you like animals? What is your favourite animal?*

The typical autistic answer is YES. Autistic women often love animals in a unique way (see the next question). Dogs, horses and cats are the animals that are mentioned most often.

2. *Do you feel a special connection with animals? Do you have the impression of mutual understanding and acceptance?*

The typical autistic answer is YES. The relationship that connects an autistic woman with her favourite(s) animal(s) is often unique and deep. They may describe this connection at a spiritual level, feeling better understood by animals than by humans and perceiving an animal's emotions better than non-autistic people, sometimes describing this as a 'sixth sense'. Temple Grandin provides an example of this special connection between an autistic woman and animals (1997).

3. *Do you relate to animals better than humans?*

This special bond can explain the deep reaction of pain and grief that autistic women experience after the death of an animal.

G. Sensory aspects and perception

1. *Do you have difficulty with tactile experiences such as wearing clothes with a rough texture and the sensation of labels and seams on your skin? When did this sensitivity start?*

The typical autistic answer is YES. It is often present since early childhood. Some autistic women have developed a greater ability to tolerate these tactile experiences, while others struggle and find them stressful every day. Some of these sensations can be specific to their gender (e.g. wearing tights, bra, make-up).

2. *Is it difficult for you to experience very light touch, such as when being greeted by people you don't know? Do you enjoy deep tactile pressure with someone you know and trust, such as a strong hug? When did this characteristic start?*

The typical autistic answer is YES. It is often present since early childhood. In general, autistic people do not like being touched by strangers, but they can appreciate a deep massage or hug that they have initiated or from specific people such as partners/children.

3. *Do you have difficulty eating some foods because of their texture? Which textures? When did this difficulty start?*

The typical autistic answer is YES. It is often present since early childhood. This may extend to even looking at people eating certain foods or thinking about a particular food. Aversive sensory experiences associated with food may be a contributary factor in developing an eating disorder.

4. *Do you have an intense perception of specific aromas? When did you start to perceive aromas in this way?*

The typical autistic answer is YES. It is often present since early childhood. Some autistic people can perceive the aromas from a specific restaurant hundreds of metres away, or be acutely aware of the aversive smell of someone's deodorant or specific cleaning products.

5. *Is it difficult for you to stay in a room with fluorescent or bright lights? Do you perceive light in an intense way? When did you start to perceive light in this way?*

The typical autistic answer is YES. It is often present since early childhood. Some autistic people have difficulty tolerating bright sunlight and intense down lights, and fluorescent lighting, which seem to flicker. There can be remarkable visual acuity, such as the ability to see specks of dust in the air or notice blemishes on a person's skin from a distance.

6. *Are you acutely aware of specific sounds and the volume of some sounds? Is it difficult for you to stay in a noisy environment? When did this difficulty start?*

The typical autistic answer is YES. It is often present since early childhood. There can be extreme distress when someone shouts, difficulty focusing on one voice when people around are talking and extraordinary auditory perception such as hearing the 'hum' of electricity in a room or the sound of a vacuum cleaner being used in another house.

Some autistic women will report having perfect pitch and it can be unbearable listening to someone sing out of tune.

7. *Do you like listening to music? Do you like the music to be very loud? Which aspect do you like most in your preferred music?*

The typical autistic answer is YES. For many autistic people, listening to their preferred music very loudly is a way to relax and relieve the tensions accumulated during the day. Some autistic women have the ability to precisely distinguish every note or voice in classical or choral music. This can lead to a career as a conductor or sound engineer.

8. *Do you have difficulty perceiving the internal sensations in your body?*

The typical autistic answer is YES. Many autistic people describe difficulties with interoception, which is the cognitive awareness of bodily sensations such as perceiving changes in heart rate, breathing or muscle tension, perceiving colour, fatigue, hunger and thirst, satiety, temperature and level of humidity, needing to go to the toilet, sexual response, etc. In some people there is almost a mind-and-body disconnect and difficulty making sense of some of the body's signals unless they are very clear and strong. This will affect the autistic person's ability to perceive and effectively regulate and communicate low levels of emotion and sensations, which seem to fly under the mental radar and may be released in an emotional meltdown or other somatic symptoms.

This lower interoceptive perception is linked to alexithymia.

9. *Do you have difficulty with manual activities and motor coordination? When did this difficulty start?*

The typical autistic answer is YES. Autism is associated with a signature profile of movement abilities. However, our clinical experience is that autistic girls and women may enjoy and excel at some manual activities and team sports more than autistic boys and men.

10. *Do you have difficulty perceiving spatial distances and/or distinguishing right from left?*

The typical autistic answer is YES. Many autistic people have a poor spatial perception, which is linked to a poor proprioception. This difficulty is frequently associated with a deficit in some executive functions such as cognitive flexibility, multitasking and decision making, and can make it difficult for some autistic people to drive a car in heavy or fast-moving traffic.

11. *Do you experience your emotions in an intense way?*

The typical autistic answer is YES. Autistic people often have hyper-emotional sensitivity, with greater internal reactions to emotional stimuli than neurotypical people. This can include an intense emotional reaction to bad news in a paper or television or a specific theme such as climate change during a conversation. Some autistic women create a mental barrier or fence to protect themselves from their intense emotional reaction.

Complementary information – Part One
Health

1. *Do you have or have you ever had sleep problems?*

The typical autistic answer is YES. It is often present since childhood. Sleep issues are frequently associated with ASD and are a concern that many autistic women share (Han *et al.* 2022).

2. *Do you have or have you ever had gastrointestinal problems?*

The typical autistic answer is YES. It is often present since early childhood (Croen *et al.* 2015).

3. *Did you or do you make use of illegal drugs?*

Some autistic women have used illegal drugs during their adolescence. Illegal drugs, misuse of prescription medication, alcohol and cannabis can be used to engage with others by reducing anxiety or to disengage from the stress and distress associated with everyday life. Autistic people have a tendency to develop addiction to a range of substances (Butwicka *et al.* 2017).

4. *Did you or do you suffer from hormonal problems and/or autoimmune conditions?*

The typical autistic answer is YES. It is often present since childhood. It is important to get a detailed description of all these problems (Croen *at al.* 2015).

General cues and indices from the interview

The clinician should pay close attention to details of the general presentation of the person that can reveal even a slight difference/oddness: clothes sense, ritualistic and soothing hand movements or motor tics during the interview, and unusual gaze behaviour. Autistic women often have more frequent and prolonged eye contact than autistic men, but there can be an unusual intensity. Many autistic women have learned over time how to use strategies to mimic and act like non-autistic people due to masking. It is important to explore whether the client's non-verbal communication abilities are contrived or stylized. The clinician may achieve this by intuition and extensive experience.

An autistic person can also have a startle reaction to sudden noises that occur during the interview (telephone, car horns or motorbikes accelerating, etc.).

There may be confirmation of the language profile associated with autism such as conversational reciprocity, switching topics rather than seeking clarification, providing too much or too little information and unusual prosody or accent.

Complementary information – Part Two

If, during the interview, the client expresses any information related to one of the following issues, it should be acknowledged and potentially further explored by a sexologist/psychologist with a strong knowledge of sexuality and ASD.

Sexuality

1. Delay in exploratory sexual behaviours

2. Questioning sexual orientation

3. History of sexual abuse

4. Boundary issues/limits regarding sexual experiences

5. Sexual promiscuity or being asexual

6. Gender flexibility, neutrality or conflict

Unfortunately, a considerable number of autistic women have experienced psychological and/or sexual violence and abuse. According to recent research, the prevalence is nearly 90 per cent (Cazalis *et al.* 2022).

ABOUT THE AUTHORS OF THE CLINICAL ASSESSMENT GUIDE

This document is the result of collaboration between several autism professionals who have combined their specific knowledge to produce the most complete clinical assessment guide possible.

Dr Isabelle Hénault and Professor Tony Attwood are both internationally renowned clinical psychologists specializing in autism and

Asperger's syndrome. It was through their daily clinical practice that they realized how it had become necessary to adapt the practices of autism diagnostic assessment for the female profile. Valentina Pasin, formerly a student under Isabelle's supervision, was able to observe numerous clinical assessment interviews based on Isabelle's and Tony's practices over a long period. Her observations were compiled to give form to this guide following advice and suggestions from clinicians. Dr Bruno Wicker, a neuroscientist by training, provided a methodology and a scientific eye to proceedings, in order to ensure the guide is well structured and accurate, taking into account current scientific research on the diagnostic assessment of adults.

Dr Isabelle Hénault is a sexologist, psychologist and director of the Clinique Autisme & Asperger de Montréal, Canada. She obtained a Master's in Sexology and a Doctorate in Psychology from the Université du Québec à Montréal. She consults privately (for individuals, couples and families) and acts as a consultant to schools and organizations. Her services also include diagnostic assessment. Isabelle gained her expertise working with people with Asperger's, especially in the domains of interpersonal relationships and sexuality. The author of a tailored socio-sexual programme, she has also collaborated on international research on sex education and psychotherapy for autistic people. She worked for more than two and a half years in Professor Attwood's clinic in Australia.

Isabelle is collaborating with Actions pour l'autisme Asperger in France. In 2005, she published *Le syndrome Asperger et la sexualité: De la puberté à l'âge adulte* [*Asperger's Syndrome and Sexuality*] (Chenelière Éducation), and is co-author of *The Autism Spectrum, Sexuality and the Law: What Every Parent and Professional Needs to Know* (Attwood, Hénault and Dubin 2014), published with Jessica Kingsley Publishers. She has also written several chapters in books on autism in Europe, the United States and Canada, and gives conference papers on these subjects as well as participating in international colloquia.

Valentina Pasin is a neuropsychologist and psychotherapist in the field of autism and other developmental conditions in Italy. She is also clinical and scientific director of a private clinic in the north of Italy, where she leads a multidisciplinary team of a dozen professionals.[2] The

---

2   www.gruppoempathie.com

team is unique in Italy, in providing diagnostic assessment services for autism, ADHD, specific learning disorders and giftedness starting from the age of six to adulthood. The team of professionals is specifically trained to provide support to clinical minorities such as females and neuroqueer people.

Valentina completed the second cycle of her Baccalauréat in Cognitive Psychology at the University of Padua, Italy, in 2010. She then completed her Master's (third cycle) in Neuroscience and Neuropsychological Rehabilitation at the University of Bologna, Italy, in 2014. She also obtained a Diploma of Higher Studies Specialized in Behavioural Interventions and interned under the supervision of Dr Hénault at the Clinique Autisme & Asperger de Montréal in 2017. She obtained the title of psychotherapist in 2023, and in the same year became professor at the SLOP (Scuola Lombarda di Psicoterapia, Lombardy School of Psychotherapy). In 2023 she won the prize 'Woman of the Year – special mention under 35' as a 'prominent female personality who, with intuition and courage, has distinguished herself by promoting initiatives that have had a particular social impact, both locally and nationally'.[3]

Professor Tony Attwood is a psychologist specializing in Asperger's syndrome. He obtained his Doctorate in Psychology from the University of London, where he was Uta Frith's student, and his Master's in Clinical Psychology from the University of Surrey, UK. He also holds an honorary rank in psychology from the University of Hull, UK.

Tony lives in Brisbane, Australia, where he is director of Attwood & Garnett Events, Brisbane, Australia, devoted to people with Asperger's. The author of numerous publications on the autism spectrum in general, and Asperger's in particular, he is popularly known as author of *The Complete Guide to Asperger's Syndrome*, which was published in 2008 and revised in 2015 by Jessica Kingsley Publishers, London.

Dr Bruno Wicker is a neuroscientist and head of research at the Centre national de la recherche scientifique (CNRS France). The author of several articles on autism, since 2014 he has devoted a large portion of his work to implementing projects that aim to improve the daily lives of autistic people, especially as regards their social and professional integration.

---

3   www.premiodonna.it

References

APA (American Psychiatric Association) (2013) *Diagnostic and Statistical Manual of Mental Disorders. Fifth Edition* (DSM-5). APA.

APA (2000) *Diagnostic and Statistical Manual of Mental Disorders. Fourth Edition, Text Revision* (DSM-IV-TR). APA.

APA (2022) *Diagnostic and Statistical Manual of Mental Disorders. Fifth Edition, Text Revision* (DSM-5-TR®). APA.

Aquilla, P. (2003) 'Sensory Issues in Individuals with Asperger Syndrome.' The Second National Conference on Asperger's Syndrome, Toronto, Ontario. Asperger's Society of Ontario.

Ariel, C. (2012) *Understanding and Connecting with Your Partner*. New Harbinger Publications.

Arnold, C. (2016) 'The invisible link between autism and anorexia.' *Spectrum*, 17 February. www.spectrumnews.org/features/deep-dive/the-invisible-link-between-autism-and-anorexia

Asperger, H. (1998) *Die «Autistischen Psychopathen» im Kindesalter. Les psychopathes autistiques pendant leur enfance*. Le Plessis-Robinson: Institut Synthélabo pour le progrès de la connaissance, [Cadillac]: L'Information psychiatrique.

Aston, M.C. (2014) *The Other Half of Asperger Syndrome (Autism Spectrum Disorder): A Guide to Living in an Intimate Relationship with a Partner Who Is on the Autism Spectrum (Second Edition)*. Jessica Kingsley Publishers.

Aston, M.C. (2003) *Aspergers in Love: Couple Relationships and Family Affairs*. Jessica Kingsley Publishers.

Attwood, T. (1998) *Asperger's Syndrome: A Guide for Parents and Professionals*. Jessica Kingsley Publishers.

Attwood, T. (2005a) *Exploring Feelings: Cognitive Behaviour Therapy to Manage Anxiety*. Future Horizons.

Attwood, T. (2005b) 'Theory of Mind and Asperger's Syndrome.' In L.J. Baker and L. Welkowitz (eds) *Asperger's Syndrome: Intervening in Schools, Clinics, and Communities* (pp.11–42). Lawrence Erlbaum Associates Publishers.

Attwood, T. (2008, revised 2015) *The Complete Guide to Asperger's Syndrome*. Jessica Kingsley Publishers.

Attwood, T. (2012) 'Girls with Asperger's syndrome: Early diagnosis is critical.' *Autism Asperger's Digest*, July–August.

Attwood, T. and Garnett, M. (2013a) *CBT to Help Young People with Asperger's Syndrome (Autism Spectrum Disorder) to Understand and Express Affection.* Jessica Kingsley Publishers.

Attwood, T. and Garnett, M. (2013b) *From Like to Love for Young People with Asperger's Syndrome (Autism Spectrum Disorder).* Jessica Kingsley Publishers.

Attwood, T. and Gray, C. (2004) 'Strategies to reduce the bullying of young children with Asperger syndrome.' *Australian Journal of Early Childhood 29*, 3, 15–23. https://doi.org/10.1177/183693910402900304

Attwood, T., Callesen, K. and Møller Nielsen, A. (2009) *The CAT-Kit: The New Cognitive Affective Training Program for Improving Communication!* Future Horizons.

Attwood, T., Garnett, M.S. and Rynkiewicz, A. (2011–17) *Questionnaire for Autism Spectrum Conditions (Q-ASC) (age 5–12 and age 13 and older).* www.mindsand-hearts.net/gq-asc-girls-questionnaire-for-autism-spectrum-condition

Attwood, T., Hénault, I. and Dubin, N. (2014) *The Autism Spectrum, Sexuality and the Law: What Every Parent and Professional Needs to Know.* Jessica Kingsley Publishers.

Auyeung, B., Allison, C., Wheelwright, S. and Baron-Cohen, S. (2012) 'Brief report: Development of the adolescent Empathy and Systematizing Quotients.' *Journal of Autism and Developmental Disorders 42*, 2225–2235. https://docs.autismre-searchcentre.com/papers/2012_Auyeung_et_al_AdolescentEQSQ_JADD.pdf

Auyeung, B., Baron-Cohen, S., Wheelwright, S. and Allison, C. (2008) 'The Autism Spectrum Quotient: Children's version (AQ-Child).' *Journal of Autism and Developmental Disorders 38*, 7, 1230–1240. doi: 10.1007/s10803-007-0504-z

Auyeung, B., Wheelwright, S., Allison, C., Atkinson, M., Samamarwickrema, N. and Baron-Cohen, S. (2009) 'The children's Empathy Quotient and Systematizing Quotient: Sex differences in typical development and in autism spectrum conditions.' *Journal of Autism and Developmental Disorders 39*, 11, 1509–1521. doi: 10.1007/s10803-009-0772-x

Barette, M.-C. (2017) 'Le syndrome d'Asperger' [television interview]. In *Deux filles le matin*, 18 January, TVA, Quebec, Canada.

Bargiela, S., Steward, R. and Mandy, W. (2016) 'The experiences of late-diagnosed women with autism spectrum conditions: An investigation of the female autism phenotype.' *Journal of Autism and Developmental Disorders 46*, 10, 3281–3294. doi: 10.1007/s10803-016-2872-8

Baron-Cohen, S. (2017) 'The eyes as window to the mind.' *The American Journal of Psychiatry 174*, 1. https://doi.org/10.1176/appi.ajp.2016.16101188

Baron-Cohen, S. (2004) *Social Stories Questionnaire* [Database record].

Baron-Cohen, S. and Wheelwright, S. (2003) 'The Friendship Questionnaire: An investigation of adults with Asperger syndrome or high-functioning autism, and normal sex differences.' *Journal of Autism and Developmental Disorders 33*, 5, 509–517. doi: 10.1023/a:1025879411971

Baron-Cohen, S. and Wheelwright, S. (2004) 'The Empathy Quotient (EQ). An investigation of adults with Asperger syndrome or high functioning autism, and normal sex differences.' *Journal of Autism and Developmental Disorders 34*, 2, 163–175. doi: 10.1023/b:jadd.0000022607.19833.0

Baron-Cohen, S., Golan, O. and Ashwin, E. (2009) 'Can emotion recognition be taught to children with autism spectrum conditions?' *Philosophical Transactions of the Royal Society B – Biological Sciences 364*, 1535, 3567–3574. doi: 10.1098/rstb.2009.0191

Baron-Cohen, S., Wheelwright, S. and Jolliffe, T. (1997) "Is there a 'language of the eyes"? Evidence from normal adults and adults with autism or Asperger syndrome.' *Visual Cognition 4*, 3, 311–331.

Baron-Cohen, S., Hoekstra, R.A., Knickmeyer, R. and Wheelwright, S. (2006) 'The Autism Spectrum Quotient (AQ) – Adolescent version.' *Journal of Autism and Developmental Disorders 36*, 3, 343–350. doi: 10.1007/s10803-006-0073-6

Baron-Cohen, S., O'Riordan, M., Stone, V., Jones, R. and Plaisted, K. (1999) 'A new test of social sensitivity: Detection of faux pas in normal children and children with Asperger syndrome.' *Journal of Autism and Developmental Disorders 29*, 407–418.

Baron-Cohen, S., Richler, J., Bisarya, D., Gurunathan, N. and Wheelwright, S. (2003) 'The systemizing quotient: An investigation of adults with Asperger syndrome or high-functioning autism, and normal sex differences.' *Philosophical Transactions of the Royal Society of London. Series B, Biological Sciences 358*, 1430, 361–374. doi: 10.1098/rstb.2002.1206

Baron-Cohen, S., Wheelwright, S., Hill, J., Raste, Y. and Plumb, I. (2001a) 'The "Reading the Mind in the Eyes" test revised version: A study with normal adults, and adults with Asperger syndrome or high-functioning autism.' *Journal of Child Psychology and Psychiatry 42*, 2, 241–252.

Baron-Cohen, S., Wheelwright, S., Skinner, R., Martin, J. and Clubley, E. (2001b) 'The Autism-Spectrum Quotient (AQ): Evidence from Asperger syndrome/high-functioning autism, males and females, scientists and mathematicians.' *Journal of Autism and Developmental Disorders 31*, 1, 5–17. doi: 10.1023/a:1005653411471

Bogdashina, O. (2012) *Questions sensorielles et perceptives dans l'autisme et le syndrome d'Asperger: Des expériences sensorielles diffférentes, des mondes perceptifs différents.* Autisme France diffusion [in French].

Brown, C.M., Attwood, T., Garnett, M. and Stokes, M.A. (2020) 'Am I autistic? Utility of the Girls Questionnaire for Autism Spectrum Condition as an autism assessment in adult women.' *Autism in Adulthood: Challenges and Management 2*, 3, 216–226. doi: 10.1089/aut.2019.0054

Butwicka, A., Långström, N., Larsson, H., Lundström, S., *et al.* (2017) 'Increased risk for substance use-related problems in autism spectrum disorders: A population-based cohort study.' *Journal of Autism and Developmental Disorders 47*, 1, 80–89. doi: 10.1007/s10803-016-2914-2

Carnes, P., Delmonico, D.L., Griffin, E., with Moriarity, J.M. (2007) *In the Shadows of the Net: Breaking Free of Compulsive Online Sexual Behavior*, 2nd edn. Hazelden Foundation.

Cazalis, F. and Lacroix, A. (2017) 'Meet Sophie, one of the many women with undiagnosed "high-functioning" autism.' The Conversation, 5 July. https://femmesautistesfrancophones.com/2017/07/21/larticle-ces-femmes-autistes-qui-signorent-republie-sur-la-chaine-de-tele-australienne-abc-news [in French].

Cazalis, F., Reyes, E., Leduc, S. and Gourion, D. (2022) 'Evidence that nine autistic women out of ten have been victims of sexual violence.' *Frontiers in Behavioral Neuroscience 16*, 852203. doi: 10.3389/fnbeh.2022.852203

Cook, B. and Garnett, M. (eds) (2018) *Spectrum Women: Walking to the Beat of Autism.* Jessica Kingsley Publishers.

Côté, S. (2016) *Favoriser l'attention par des stratégies sensorielles.* Chenelière Éducation [in French].

Croen, L.A., Zerbo, O., Qian, Y., Massolo, M.L., *et al.* (2015) 'The health status of adults on the autism spectrum.' *Autism 19,* 7, 814823. https://doi.org/10.1177/1362361315577517

Dachez, J. (2020) *Invisible Differences: A Story of Asperger's, Adulting, and Living a Life in Full Color.* Oni Press.

Davidson, J. and Tamas, S. (2016) 'Autism and the ghost of gender.' *Emotion, Space and Society 19,* 59–65. https://doi.org/10.1016/j.emospa.2015.09.009

Derogatis, L.R. and Melisaratos, N. (1982) *Synopsis of the Derogatis Sexual Functioning Inventory (DSFI).* www.derogatis-tests.com

Edmonds, G. and Worton, D. (2005) *The Asperger Love Guide: A Practical Guide for Adults with Asperger's Syndrome to Seeking, Establishing and Maintaining Successful Relationships.* SAGE Publications.

Eivors, A. and Nesbitt, S. (2005) *Hunger for Understanding: A Workbook for Helping Young People to Understand and Overcome Anorexia Nervosa.* John Wiley & Sons.

Ekman, P. (2003) *Emotions Revealed: Recognizing Faces and Feelings to Improve Communication and Emotional Life.* Times Books/Henry Holt & Co.

Foreman, J. (2003) 'A look at empathy, please!' *The Boston Globe.*

Frith, U. (ed.) (1991) *Autism and Asperger Syndrome.* Cambridge University Press.

Gabor, D. (2011) *How to Start a Conversation and Make Friends.* Touchstone.

Garnett, M. and Attwood, T. (2021) *Autism Working: A Seven-Stage Plan to Thriving at Work.* Jessica Kingsley Publishers.

Gillberg, C. (2018) 'Are autism and anorexia nervosa related?' *The British Journal of Psychiatry 142,* 4, 428 [letter]. www.cambridge.org/core/journals/the-british-journal-of-psychiatry/article/are-autism-and-anorexia-nervosa-related/8802FFF186F0AF79995D8CB9F250D085

Goetz, T.G. (2023) *Gender Is Really Strange.* Jessica Kingsley Publishers.

Goldenfeld, N., Baron-Cohen, S. and Wheelwright, S., (2005) 'Empathizing and systemizing in males, females, and autism.' *Clinical Neuropsychiatry 2,* 6, 338–345.

Grandin, T. (1995) *Thinking in Pictures: And Other Reports from My Life with Autism.* Doubleday.

Grandin, T. (1997) 'Thinking the way animals do: Unique insights from a person with a singular understanding.' Western Horseman, 140–145. www.grandin.com/references/thinking.animals.html

Grandin, T. and Panek, R. (2013) *The Autistic Brain: Helping Different Kinds of Minds Succeed.* Houghton Mifflin Harcourt.

Grandin, T. and Panek, R. (2014) *The Autistic Brain: Exploring the Strength of a Different Kind of Mind.* Rider.

Gray, S., Ruble, L. and Dalrymple, N. (1996) *Autism and Sexuality: A Guide for Instruction.* Autism Society of Indiana.

Griffiths, D., Richards, D., Fedoroff, P. and Watson, S.L. (2002) *Ethical Dilemmas: Sexuality and Developmental Disability.* NADD Press.

Guerrero, L. (2013) *Lundi, je vais être Luka.* Bayard Canada.

Han, G.T., Trevisan, D.A., Abel, E.A., Cummings, E.M., *et al.* (2022) 'Associations between sleep problems and domains relevant to daytime functioning and clinical symptomatology in autism: A meta-analysis.' *Autism Research 15,* 7, 1249–1260. https://doi.org/10.1002/aur.2758

Happé, F.G.E. (1994) 'An advanced test of theory of mind: Understanding of story characters' thoughts and feelings by able autistic, mentally handicapped, and normal children and adults.' *Journal of Autism and Developmental Disorders 24*, 129–154. https://link.springer.com/article/10.1007/BF02172093

Haracopos, D. and Pedersen, L. (1999) *The Danish Report*. Autism Independent UK.

Le HAS (Haute autorité de santé) (2011) 'Recommandation de bonne pratique. Autisme et autres troubles envahissants du développement: diagnostic et évaluation chez l'adulte.' www.has-sante.fr/portail/upload/docs/application/pdf/2011-10/autisme_et_autres_ted_diagnostic_et_evaluation_chez_ladulte_-_recommandations.pdf

Hayden, T. (1980) *One Child*. HarperElement.

Hellemans, H. and Deboutte, D. (2002) 'Autism spectrum disorder and sexuality.' Paper presented at the Inaugural World Autism Congress, Melbourne, 10–14 November.

Hénault, I. (2005) *Asperger's Syndrome and Sexuality: From Adolescence through Adulthood*. Jessica Kingsley Publishers.

Hénault, I. and Attwood, T. (2002) 'The Sexual Profile of Adults with Asperger Syndrome: The Need for Comprehension, Support and Education.' Paper presented at the World First Autism Congress, Melbourne.

Hendrickx, S. (2008) *Love, Sex and Long-Term Relationships: What People with Asperger Syndrome Really Want*. Jessica Kingsley Publishers.

Holliday Willey, L. (2014) *Pretending to Be Normal: Living with Asperger's Syndrome (Autism Spectrum Disorder) (Expanded Edition)*. Jessica Kingsley Publishers.

Howlin, P., Baron-Cohen, S. and Hadwin, J.A. (1999) *Teaching Children with Autism to Mind-Read*. John Wiley & Sons.

Hull, L., Mandy, W., Lai, M.-C., Baron-Cohen, S., *et al.* (2019) 'Development and validation of the Camouflaging Autistic Traits Questionnaire (CAT-Q).' *Journal of Autism and Developmental Disorders 49*, 3, 819–833. doi: 10.1007/s10803-018-3792-6

Hull, L., Petrides, K.V., Allison, C., Smith, P., *et al.* (2017) '"Putting on my best normal": Social camouflaging in adults with autism spectrum conditions.' *Journal of Autism and Developmental Disorders 47*, 8, 2519–2534. doi: 10.1007/s10803-017-3166-5

Israel, G.E. and Tarver II, D.E. (1997) *Transgender Care: Recommended Guidelines, Practical Information & Personal Accounts*. Temple University Press.

Jones, R.M., Wheelwright, S., Farrell, K., Martin, E., *et al.* (2012) 'Brief report: Female-to-male transsexual people and autistic traits.' *Journal of Autism and Developmental Disorders 42*, 2, 301–306. doi: 10.1007/s10803-011-1227-8.

Kana, R.K., Libero, L.E. and Moore, M.S. (2011) 'Disrupted cortical connectivity theory as an explanatory model for autism spectrum disorders.' *Physics of Life Reviews 8*, 410–437.

Kanner, L. (1943) 'Autistic disturbances of affective contact.' *Nervous Child 2*, 217–250.

Kopp, S. and Gillberg, C. (2011) 'The Autism Spectrum Screening Questionnaire (ASSQ)-Revised Extended Version (ASSQ-REV): An instrument for better capturing the autism phenotype in girls? A preliminary study involving 191 clinical cases and community controls.' *Research in Developmental Disabilities 32*, 6, 2875–2888. doi: 10.1016/j.ridd.2011.05.017

Kourti, M. (2021) *Working with Autistic Transgender and Non-Binary People: Research, Practice and Experience*. Jessica Kingsley Publishers.

Kourti, M. and MacLeod, A. (2019) '"I don't feel like a gender, I feel like myself": Autistic individuals raised as girls exploring gender identity.' *Autism in Adulthood 1*, 1, 52–59. doi: 10.1089/aut.2018.0001

Lai, M.-C. and Baron-Cohen, S. (2015) 'Identifying the lost generation of adults with autism spectrum conditions.' *The Lancet. Psychiatry 2*, 11, 1013–1027. doi: 10.1016/S2215-0366(15)00277-1

Langmann, A., Becker, J., Poustka, L. and Becker, K. (2017) 'Diagnostic utility of the autism diagnostic observation schedule in a clinical sample of adolescents and adults.' *Research in Autism Spectrum Disorders 34*, 34–43.

Lawrence, E.J., Shaw, P., Baker, D., Baron-Cohen, S. and David, A.S. (2004) 'Measuring empathy: Reliability and validity of the Empathy Quotient.' *Psychological Medicine 34*, 5, 911–924. doi: 10.1017/s0033291703001624

Lawson, W. (2003) 'Foreword.' In O. Bogdashina, *Sensory Perceptual Issues in Autism and Asperger Syndrome*. Jessica Kingsley Publishers.

Lebrun, S. (2015) *L'autisme apprivoisé*. Olographes.

Lewis, L.F. (2017) 'A mixed methods study of barriers to formal diagnosis of autism spectrum disorder in adults.' *Journal of Autism and Developmental Disorders 47*, 8, 2410–2424. doi: 10.1007/s10803-017-3168-3

Loomes, R., Hull, L., Polmear, W. and Mandy, L. (2017) 'What is the male-to-female ratio in autism spectrum disorder? A systematic review and meta-analysis.' *Journal of the American Academy of Child and Adolescent Psychiatry 56*, 6, 466–474. doi: 10.1016/j.jaac.2017.03.013

Mandy, W. and Steward, R. (2016) 'Women with autism hide complex struggles behind masks.' *Autism Research News*, 20 September. www.spectrumnews.org/opinion/viewpoint/women-autism-hide-complex-struggles-behind-masks

Martin, A. (2010) *La crypte cassée: Essai sur l'écriture posttraumatique*. Liber Editions.

Martin, V. (2011) 'Vivre et créer avec le syndrome d'Asperger.' *Journal L'UQAM XXXVIII*, 6. www.actualites.uqam.ca/2011/vivre-et-creer-avec-le-syndrome-dasperger

MAtv (2015) 'L'autisme autrement. 2. L'anxiété' [Vidéo]. https://matv.ca/montreal/mes-emissions/l-autisme-autrement

May, A. [Martin, Annyck] (2017) 'Autisme Asperger, un diagnostic à l'âge adulte?' *Regard9*, 19 April. www.regard9.ca/blogueR9/2017/04/autisme-asperger-diagnostic-adulte

McKibbin, K. (2015) *Life on the Autism Spectrum. A Guide for Girls and Women*. Jessica Kingsley Publishers.

Milton, D. (2012) 'On the ontological status of autism: The "double empathy problem".' *Disability and Society 27*, 3, 883–887.

Mitchell, P., Cassidy, S. and Sheppard, E. (2019) 'The double empathy problem, camouflage, and the value of expertise from experience.' *Behavioral and Brain Sciences 42*, 33–34. https://doi.org/10.1017/S0140525X18002212

Moore, M. (2023) 'Are there differences between autistic boys and girls?' PsychCentral, 17 October. https://psychcentral.com/autism/comparison-of-boys-and-girls-living-with-autism-spectrum-disorder

Moreno, S., Wheeler, M. and Parkinson, K. (2012) *The Partner's Guide to Asperger Syndrome*. Jessica Kingsley Publishers.

Ormond, S., Brownlow, C., Garnett, M.S., Rynkiewicz, A. and Attwood, T. (2018) 'Profiling autism symptomatology: An exploration of the Q-ASC parental report scale in capturing sex differences in autism.' *Journal of Autism and Developmental Disorders 48*, 2, 389–403. doi: 10.1007/s10803-017-3324-9

Ostrolenk, A. (2017) 'Quand les enfants autistes lisent avant de parler.' *Sur Le Spectre*. http://grouperecherautismemontreal.ca/Documents/Quand%20les%20enfants%20autistes%20olisent%20avant%20de%20parler.pdf

Ostrolenk, A., Forgeot d'Arc, B., Jelenic, P., Samson, F., & Mottron, L. (2017) 'Hyperlexia: Systematic review, neurocognitive modelling, and outcome.' *Neuroscience and Biobehavioral Review, 79*, 134–149. doi: 10.1016/j.neubiorev.2017.04.029

Ouellette, A. (2011) 'Causerie avec Antoine Ouellette pour la parution de l'essai Musique autiste chez Tryptique, 27 octobre, à la Librairie Monet' [Video]. https://youtu.be/yWDOt1aCqdY

Ouellette, A. (2018) *Musique autiste: Vivre et composer avec le syndrome d'Asperger*. Varia (Editions).

Ouimet, M. (2017) 'Je suis une adulte et il m'arrive encore de faire des crises!' ['I am an adult and I still get meltdowns!'] HuffPost, 14 June. www.huffpost.com/archive/qc/entry/je-suis-une-adulte-et-il-marrive-encore-de-faire-des-crises_b_10397802 [in French].

Overholser, J.C. (1996) 'Cognitive-behavioral treatment of depression, part V: Enhancing self-esteem and self-control.' *Journal of Contemporary Psychotherapy 26*, 163–176.

Poulin, M.-H. (2015) 'Communiquer un sens à la fois' [Video for Parle-moi de TSA!]. www.facebook.com/1642729429313592/videos/166713187354001

Quintas, E., with Fourcade, M.-B. and Pronovost, M., translated by Roth, K. (2015) *Cultural Mediation: Questions and Answers*. Culture pour tous.

Ritvo, R.A., Ritvo, E.R., Guthrie, D., Ritvo, M.J., *et al*. (2011) 'The Ritvo Autism Asperger Diagnostic Scale–Revised (RAADS–R): A scale to assist the diagnosis of autism spectrum disorder in adults: An international validation study.' *Journal of Autism and Developmental Disorders 41*, 8, 1076–1089. doi: 10.1007/s10803-010-1133-5

Rynkiewicz, A., Schuller, B., Marchi, E., Piana, S., Camurri, A., Lassalle, A. and Baron-Cohen, S. (2016) 'An investigation of the "female camouflage effect" in autism using a computerized ADOS-2 test and a test of sex/gender differences.' *Molecular Autism 7*, 10, 1–8. https://docs.autismresearchcentre.com/papers/2016_Rynkiewicz_MolecularAutism_Female_camouflage-effect.pdf

Sandin, S., Lichtenstein, P., Kuja-Halkola, R., Hultman, C., Larsson, H. and Reichenberg, A. (2017) 'The heritability of autism spectrum disorder.' *Journal of the American Medical Association 318*, 12, 1182–1184. doi: 10.1001/jama.2017.12141

Simone, R. (2010) *Aspergirls: Empowering females with Asperger Syndrome*. Jessica Kingsley Publishers.

Simone, R. (2013) *L'Asperger au féminin. Comment favoriser l'autonomie des femmes atteintes du syndrome d'Asperger*. De Boeck.

Smith Myles, B., Topscott Cook, K., Miller, N.E., Rinner, L. and Robbins, L.A. (2001) *Asperger Syndrome and Sensory Issues: Practical Solutions for Making Sense of the World*. Autism Asperger Publishing Co.

Stewart, C.S., McEwen, F.S., Konstantellou, A., Eisler, I. and Simic, M. (2017) 'Impact of ASD traits on treatment outcomes of eating disorders in girls.' *European Eating Disorders Review 25*, 2, 123–128. https://doi.org/10.1002/erv.2497

Stone, V.E., Baron-Cohen, S. and Knight, R.T. (1998) 'Frontal lobe contributions to theory of mind.' *Journal of Cognitive Neuroscience 10*, 5, 640–656. doi: 10.1162/089892998562942

Strang, J.F., Meagher, H., Kenworthy, L., de Vries, A.L.C., *et al.* (2018) 'Initial clinical guidelines for co-occurring autism spectrum disorder and gender dysphoria or incongruence in adolescents.' *Journal of Clinical Child and Adolescent Psychology 47*, 1, 105–115. doi: 10.1080/15374416.2016.1228462

Taillefer, L., Hénault, I., Langlois, L., Pommier, C. and Prévost, M.-J. (2015) 'Lignes directrices en matière de sexualité pour les personnes présentant une déficience intellectuelle (DI) ou une DI et un trouble du spectre de l'autisme (TSA).' ['Guidelines on the sexual lives of hospitalized patients in the IUSMM Intellectual Disability Psychiatry Program']. Institut universitaire en santé mentale de Montréal. https://numerique.banq.qc.ca/patrimoine/details/52327/2497192

Tavassoli, T., Hoekstra, R.A. and Baron-Cohen, S. (2014) 'The Sensory Perception Quotient (SPQ): Development and validation of a new sensory questionnaire for adults with and without autism.' *Molecular Autism 5*, 29. www.molecularautism.com/content/5/1/29

Westwood, H. and Tchanturia, K. (2017) 'Autism spectrum disorder in anorexia nervosa: An updated literature review.' *Current Psychiatry Reports 19*, 7, 41. doi: 10.1007/s11920-017-0791-9

Wheelwright, S., Baron-Cohen, S., Goldenfeld, N., Delaney, J., *et al.* (2006) 'Predicting Autism Spectrum Quotient (AQ) from the Systemizing Quotient-Revised (SQ-R) and Empathy Quotient (EQ).' *Brain Research 1079*, 1, 47–56. doi: 10.1016/j.brainres.2006.01.012

WHO (World Health Organization) (1993) *The ICD-10 Classification of Mental and Behavioural Disorders: Clinical Descriptions and Diagnostic Guidelines.* www.who.int/docs/default-source/classification/other-classifications/bluebook.pdf?sfvrsn=374758f7_2

WHO (2019/2021) *International Classification of Diseases, Eleventh Revision* (ICD-11). https://icd.who.int/browse/2024-01/mms/en

Wicker, B., Fonlupt, P., Hubert, B., Tardif, C., Gepner, B. and Deruelle, C. (2008) 'Abnormal cerebral effective connectivity during explicit emotional processing in adults with autism spectrum disorder.' *Social Cognitive and Affective Neuroscience 3*, 3, 135–143. doi: 10.1093/scan/nsn007.

Willey, L.H. (2001) *Asperger in the Family: Redefining Normal.* Jessica Kingsley Publishers.

Willey, L.H. (1999) *Pretending to Be Normal: Living with Asperger's Syndrome (Autism Spectrum Disorder).* Jessica Kingsley Publishers.

Willey, L.H. (2011) *Safety Skills for Asperger Women: How to Save a Perfectly Good Female Life.* Jessica Kingsley Publishers.

Wing, L. (1981) 'Asperger's syndrome: A clinical account.' *Psychological Medicine 11*, 1, 115–129. https://doi.org/10.1017/S0033291700053332

Wiskerke, J., Stern, H. and Igelström, K.M. (2018) 'Camouflaging of repetitive movements in autistic female and transgender adults.' *BioRxiv.* www.dx.doi.org/10.1101/412619

Woodbury-Smith, M.R., Robinson, J., Wheelwright, S. and Baron-Cohen, S. (2005) 'Screening adults for Asperger syndrome using the AQ: A preliminary study of its diagnostic validity in clinical practice.' *Journal of Autism and Developmental Disorders 35*, 3, 331–335. doi: 10.1007/s10803-005-3300-7

Zeliadt, N. (2018) 'Les filles autistes ont un risque élevé de subir des violences sexuelles, selon une vaste étude.' www.femmesautistesfrancophones.

com/2018/05/22/les-filles-autistes-ont-un-risque-eleve-detre-abusees-sexuellement-selon-une-vaste-etude [in French].

Zucker, N. (2015) 'Girls with autism may stop eating to blunt social pain.' *Transmitter*, 19 October. www.spectrumnews.org/opinion/girls-with-autism-may-stop-eating-to-blunt-social-pain

FURTHER READING

Attwood, T. and Grandin, T. (2006) *Asperger's and Girls: World-Renowned Experts Join Those with Asperger's Syndrome to Resolve Issues that Girls and Women Face Every Day!* Future Horizons.

Autism Spectrum Australia (Aspect) (2017) 'Girls and women on the Autism Spectrum.' www.autismspectrum.org.au

Baldwin, S. and Costley, D. (2016) 'The experiences and needs of female adults with high-functioning autism spectrum disorder.' *Autism 20*, 4, 483–495.

Cridland, E.K., Jones, S.C., Caputi, P. and Magee, C.A. (2014) 'Being a girl in a boys' world: Investigating the experiences of girls with autism spectrum disorders during adolescence.' *Journal of Autism and Developmental Disorders 44*, 6, 1261–1274.

Dworzynsky, K., Ronald, A., Bolton, P. and Happé, F. (2012) 'How different are girls and boys above and below the diagnostic threshold for autism spectrum disorders?' *Journal of the American Academy of Child and Adolescent Psychiatry 51*, 8, 788–797.

Gould, J. and Ashton-Smith, J. (2011) 'Missed diagnosis or misdiagnosis? Girls and women on the autism spectrum.' *Good Autism Practice 12*, 1, 34–41.

Grandin, T. and Barron, S. (2005) *The Unwritten Rules of Social Relationships*. Future Horizons.

Hartley, S.L. and Sikora, D.M. (2009) 'Sex differences in autism spectrum disorder: An examination of developmental functioning, autistic symptoms, and coexisting behavior problems in toddlers.' *Journal of Autism and Developmental Disorders 39*, 12, 1715.

Hendrickx, S. (2015) *Women and Girls with Autism Spectrum Disorder: Understanding Life Experiences from Early Childhood to Old Age*. Jessica Kingsley Publishers.

Kanfiszer, L., Davies, F. and Collins, S. (2017) '"I was just so different": The experiences of women diagnosed with an autism spectrum disorder in adulthood in relation to gender and social relationships.' *Autism*, 1362361316687987.

Kirkovski, M., Enticott, P.G. and Fitzgerald, P.B. (2013) 'A review of the role of female gender in autism spectrum disorders.' *Journal of Autism and Developmental Disorders 43*, 11, 2584–603.

Lai, M.C., Lombardo, M.V., *et al.* (2013) 'Biological sex affects the neurobiology of autism.' *Brain 136*, 9, 2799–2815.

Nichols, S. (2009) *Girls Growing up on the Autism Spectrum: What Parents and Professionals Should Know about the Pre-Teen and Teenagers Years*. Jessica Kingsley Publishers.

APPENDICES

*

Questionnaire for the Diagnostic Assessment of Autism in Females (QDAAF)

Protocol 1

TONY ATTWOOD, ISABELLE HÉNAULT,
VALENTINA PASIN AND BRUNO WICKER

Name:. . . . .

Surname: . . . .

Date of birth: . . . . . / . . . . . / . . . . .

Today's date: . . . . . / . . . . . / . . . . .

Other personal information:

. . . .

. . . .

. . . .

. . . .

. . . .

. . . .

. . . .

. . . .

∗

Previous diagnosis:

- ☐ Depression
- ☐ Borderline personality disorder
- ☐ Bipolar disorder
- ☐ Anorexia or eating disorders
- ☐ Anxiety and/or panic attack
- ☐ Social phobia
- ☐ Avoidant personality
- ☐ Burnout
- ☐ Other(s): . . . .
- ☐ None

Past medication:

. . . .

. . . .

. . . .

Present medication:

. . . .

. . . .

. . . .

Health:

- ☐ Sleeping problems
- ☐ Gastrointestinal problems
- ☐ Hormonal problems
- ☐ Autoimmune conditions
- ☐ Drug addiction

Notes:

. . . .

. . . .

. . . .

A	**Self-recognition as autistic**
A.1	When was the first time you learned about autism?
A.2	Do you recognize yourself in some aspects of what you have heard/read about autism? If yes, describe in what way.
A.3	Did you ever think you were different from children your age? If yes, when did you start having these thoughts, and how did you perceive yourself as different?
B	**Childhood and school years**
B.1	What memories do you have about your primary school and secondary school years?
B.2	What memories do you have about being a student at college and/or university?
B.3	Was it difficult to make friends? And now?
B.4	How many friends did you have? And now?
B.5	Did you have an imaginary friend? And have one now?
B.6	Have you ever been the victim of bullying and teasing?
B.7	Did you observe other children rather than talk and interact with them?
B.8	Did you like to watch films, soap operas or television series to observe and study the characters' social behaviours and interactions?
B.9	Did you have one or more people/characters that you used as models of behaviours?
B.10	Were you a child who preferred to be alone and being in your imaginary world?
B.11	Did you try to interact with girls of your age and become friends but frequently without success?
B.12	Did you experience episodes of situational mutism as a child or adolescent? And now?
B.13	Have you ever been interested in boys (or any other kind of romantic relationships)? If yes, when did you start?
B.14	What kind of hobbies did you have when you were a child? And now?

C	**Social interactions**
C.1	Is it difficult for you to participate in activities with many people (group activities, meetings, events, hanging out with a large group of friends or colleagues, etc.)?
C.2	Do you feel exhausted mentally and physically after a day/some hours just surrounded by many people?
C.3	After a day/some hours surrounded by many people, do you feel the need to be alone and do your favourite activity?
C.4	Do you experience some difficulties following a conversation with two or more people?
C.5	Is it difficult for you to understand the emotional reactions of others?
C.6	Do people close to you (family, friends, partner, etc.) sometimes tell you that you have a too intense reaction to a particular situation?
C.7	Is it very difficult for you to have a superficial conversation (social chit-chat) or to talk about general topics (the weather, politics, sport, gossip, etc.)?
C.8	Do you feel like you are practising the social rules and conventions in an unnatural, not spontaneous, way?
C.9	Is it a problem for you to understand when and/or how to stop a conversation?
C.10	Do you find it difficult to talk by phone when you cannot see the other person and their reactions?
C.11	Is it difficult for you to take notes during a conversation on the phone?
D	**Cognitive aspects**
D.1	Do you think in pictures? Are you a visual thinker?
D.2	Do you tend to see patterns and notice systems more than other people?
D.3	Do you have exceptional long-term memory with details or information that attracts your attention (or connected to your special interest)?
D.4	For you, is everything 'black or white'?
D.5	Are you a perfectionist? Are you able to find errors where other people can't?
D.6	Do you feel the need to live and work in an organized and structured environment? Do you feel anxious if your order is changed by someone?
D.7	Do you have set routines in your daily life? What happens if something or someone changes your routine?
D.8	Are you an honest but also naive person?

D.9	Is it difficult for you to read between the lines in a conversation?
D.10	Do you understand what people say in a literal way?
D.11	Is it very difficult for you to tell lies?
D.12	Do you feel your mind is full of feelings, thoughts or images? Is it difficult for you to translate them into words?
D.13	Do you feel like your mind is always working, even during the night?
D.14	Is it difficult for you to remember spoken instructions?
D.15	Do you like to deeply understand what you are interested in to precisely understand how things work, to always learn new things and explore them till the moment you feel you have totally understood them?
E	**Relationships**
E.1	Do you use different masks or characters in various situations in your everyday life?
E.2	Do people close to you (family, friends, partner, etc.) say that you are too direct and without filters, but according to your perspective, you are just telling the truth?
E.3	In your general experiences, are you attracted to people with a strong personality?
E.4	In your relationships, are you attracted to a person rather than his/her/their gender?
F	**Animals**
F.1	Do you like the animals? What is your favourite animal?
F.2	Do you feel a special connection with animals? Do you have the impression of mutual understanding and acceptance?
F.3	Do you relate to animals better than humans?
G	**Sensory aspects and perception**
G.1	Do you have difficulty with tactile experiences such as wearing clothes with a rough texture and the sensation of labels and seams on your skin? When did this sensitivity start?
G.2	Is it difficult for you to experience very light touch, such as when being greeted by people you don't know? Do you enjoy deep tactile pressure with someone you know and trust, such as a strong hug? When did this characteristic start?
G.3	Do you have difficulty eating some foods because of their texture? Which textures? When did this difficulty start?
G.4	Do you have an intense perception of specific aromas? When did you start to perceive aromas in this way?

G.5	Is it difficult for you to stay in a room with fluorescent or bright lights? Do you perceive light in an intense way? When did you start to perceive light in this way?
G.6	Are you acutely aware of specific sounds and the volume of some sounds? Is it difficult for you to stay in a noisy environment? When did this difficulty start?
G.7	Do you like listening to music? Do you like the music to be very loud? Which aspect do you like most in your preferred music?
G.8	Do you have difficulty perceiving the internal sensations in your body?
G.9	Do you have difficulty with manual activities and motor coordination? When did this difficulty start?
G.10	Do you have difficulty perceiving spatial distances and/or distinguishing right from left?
G.11	Do you experience your emotions in an intense way?
H	**Health**
H.1	Do you have or have you ever had sleep problems?
H.2	Do you have or have you ever had gastrointestinal problems?
H.3	Did you or do you make use of drugs?
H.4	Did you or do you suffer from hormonal problems and/or autoimmune conditions?
I	**Sexuality**
I.1	Delay in exploratory sexual behaviours
I.2	Questioning sexual orientation
I.3	History of sexual abuse
I.4	Boundary issues/limits regarding sexual experiences
I.5	Sexual promiscuity or being asexual
I.6	Gender flexibility, neutrality or conflict

*

Questionnaire for the Diagnostic Assessment of Autism in Females (QDAAF)

Protocol 2

TONY ATTWOOD, ISABELLE HÉNAULT, VALENTINA PASIN AND BRUNO WICKER

Name:. . . . .

Surname: . . . .

Date of birth: . . . . . / . . . . . / . . . . .

Today's date: . . . . . / . . . . . / . . . . .

Other personal information:

. . . .

. . . .

. . . .

. . . .

. . . .

. . . .

. . . .

. . . .

*

Previous diagnosis:

- ☐ Depression
- ☐ Borderline personality disorder
- ☐ Bipolar disorder
- ☐ Anorexia or eating disorders
- ☐ Anxiety and/or panic attack
- ☐ Social phobia
- ☐ Avoidant personality
- ☐ Burnout
- ☐ Other(s): . . . .
- ☐ None

Past medication:

. . . .

. . . .

. . . .

Present medication:

. . . .

. . . .

. . . .

Health:

- ☐ Sleeping problems
- ☐ Gastrointestinal problems
- ☐ Hormonal problems
- ☐ Autoimmune conditions
- ☐ Drug addiction

Notes:

. . . .

. . . .

. . . .

A. Self-recognition as autistic

1. When was the first time you learned about autism?

    . . . .

    . . . .

    . . . .

    . . . .

    . . . .

2. Do you recognize yourself in some aspects of what you have heard/
    read about autism? If yes, describe in what way.

    . . . .

    . . . .

    . . . .

    . . . .

    . . . .

3. Did you ever think you were different from children your age? If yes,
    when did you start having these thoughts, and how did you perceive
    yourself as different?

    . . . .

    . . . .

    . . . .

    . . . .

    . . . .

B. Childhood and school years

1. What memories do you have about your primary school and secondary school years?

    . . . .

    . . . .

    . . . .

    . . . .

    . . . .

2. What memories do you have about being a student at college and/or university?

    . . . .

    . . . .

    . . . .

    . . . .

    . . . .

3. Was it difficult to make friends? And now?

    . . . .

    . . . .

    . . . .

    . . . .

    . . . .

4. How many friends did you have? And now?

    . . . .

    . . . .

    . . . .

    . . . .

    . . . .

5. Did you have an imaginary friend? And have one now?

. . . .

. . . .

. . . .

. . . .

. . . .

6. Have you ever been the victim of bullying and teasing?

. . . .

. . . .

. . . .

. . . .

. . . .

7. Did you observe other children rather than talk and interact with them?

. . . .

. . . .

. . . .

. . . .

. . . .

8. Did you like to watch films, soap operas or television series to observe and study the characters' social behaviours and interactions?

. . . .

. . . .

. . . .

. . . .

. . . .

9. Did you have one or more people/characters that you used as models of behaviours?

. . . .

. . . .

. . . .

. . . .

. . . .

10. Were you a child who preferred to be alone and being in your imaginary world?

. . . .

. . . .

. . . .

. . . .

. . . .

11. Did you try to interact with girls of your age and become friends but frequently without success?

. . . .

. . . .

. . . .

. . . .

. . . .

12. Did you experience some episodes of situational mutism as a child or adolescent? And now?

. . . .

. . . .

. . . .

. . . .

. . . .

13. Have you ever been interested in boys (or any other kind of romantic relationships)? If yes, when did you start?

. . . .

. . . .

. . . .

. . . .

. . . .

14. What kind of hobbies did you have when you were a child? And now?

. . . .

. . . .

. . . .

. . . .

. . . .

C. Social interactions

1. Is it difficult for you to participate in activities with many people (group activities, meetings, events, hanging out with a large group of friends or colleagues, etc.)?

. . . .

. . . .

. . . .

. . . .

. . . .

2. Do you feel exhausted mentally and physically after a day/some hours just surrounded by many people?

. . . .

. . . .

. . . .

. . . .

✱

3. After a day/some hours surrounded by many people, do you feel the need to be alone and do your favourite activity?

....

....

....

....

....

4. Do you experience some difficulties following a conversation with two or more people?

....

....

....

....

....

5. Is it difficult for you to understand the emotional reactions of others?

....

....

....

....

....

6. Do people close to you (family, friends, partner, etc.) sometimes tell you that you have a too intense reaction to a particular situation?

....

....

....

....

....

7. Is it very difficult for you to have a superficial conversation (social chit-chat) or to talk about general topics (the weather, politics, sport, gossip, etc.)?

. . . .

. . . .

. . . .

. . . .

. . . .

8. Do you feel like you are practising the social rules and conventions in an unnatural, not spontaneous, way?

. . . .

. . . .

. . . .

. . . .

. . . .

9. Is it a problem for you to understand when and/or how to stop a conversation?

. . . .

. . . .

. . . .

. . . .

. . . .

10. Do you find it difficult to talk by phone when you cannot see the other person and their reactions?

. . . .

. . . .

. . . .

. . . .

11. Is it difficult for you to take notes during a conversation on the phone?

....

....

....

....

....

D. Cognitive aspects

1. Do you think in pictures? Are you a visual thinker?

....

....

....

....

....

2. Do you tend to see patterns and notice systems more than other people?

....

....

....

....

....

3. Do you have exceptional long-term memory with details or information that attracts your attention (or connected to your special interest)?

....

....

....

....

4. For you, is everything 'black or white'?

. . . .

. . . .

. . . .

. . . .

. . . .

5. Are you a perfectionist? Are you able to find errors where other people can't?

. . . .

. . . .

. . . .

. . . .

. . . .

6. Do you feel the need to live and work in an organized and structured environment? Do you feel anxious if your order is changed by someone?

. . . .

. . . .

. . . .

. . . .

. . . .

7. Do you have set routines in your daily life? What happens if something or someone changes your routine?

. . . .

. . . .

. . . .

. . . .

. . . .

8. Are you an honest but also naive person?

. . . .

. . . .

. . . .

. . . .

. . . .

9. Is it difficult for you to read between the lines in a conversation?

. . . .

. . . .

. . . .

. . . .

. . . .

10. Do you understand what people say in a literal way?

. . . .

. . . .

. . . .

. . . .

. . . .

11. Is it very difficult for you to tell lies?

. . . .

. . . .

. . . .

. . . .

. . . .

*

12. Do you feel your mind is full of feelings, thoughts or images? Is it difficult for you to translate them into words?

. . . .

. . . .

. . . .

. . . .

. . . .

13. Do you feel like your mind is always working, even during the night?

. . . .

. . . .

. . . .

. . . .

. . . .

14. Is it difficult for you to remember spoken instructions?

. . . .

. . . .

. . . .

. . . .

. . . .

15. Do you like to deeply understand what you are interested in, to precisely understand how things work, to always learn new things and explore them till the moment you feel you have totally understood them?

. . . .

. . . .

. . . .

. . . .

. . . .

$*$

E. Relationships

1. Do you use different masks or characters in various situations in your everyday life?

    . . . .

    . . . .

    . . . .

    . . . .

    . . . .

2. Do people close to you (family, friends, partner, etc.) say that you are too direct and without filters, but according to your perspective, you are just telling the truth?

    . . . .

    . . . .

    . . . .

    . . . .

    . . . .

3. In your general experiences, are you attracted to people with a strong personality?

    . . . .

    . . . .

    . . . .

    . . . .

    . . . .

4. In your relationships, are you attracted to a person rather than his/her/their gender?

    . . . .

    . . . .

    . . . .

*

. . . .

. . . .

F. Animals

1. Do you like animals? What is your favourite animal?

. . . .

. . . .

. . . .

. . . .

. . . .

2. Do you feel a special connection with animals? Do you have the impression of mutual understanding and acceptance?

. . . .

. . . .

. . . .

. . . .

. . . .

3. Do you relate to animals better than humans?

. . . .

. . . .

. . . .

. . . .

. . . .

G. Sensory aspects and perception

1. Do you have difficulty with tactile experiences such as wearing clothes with a rough texture and the sensation of labels and seams on your skin? When did this sensitivity start?

. . . .

....
....
....
....

2. Is it difficult for you to experience very light touch, such as when being greeted by people you don't know? Do you enjoy deep tactile pressure with someone you know and trust, such as a strong hug? When did this characteristic start?

....
....
....
....
....

3. Do you have difficulty eating some foods because of their texture? Which textures? When did this difficulty start?

....
....
....
....
....

4. Do you have an intense perception of specific aromas? When did you start to perceive aromas in this way?

....
....
....
....
....

5. Is it difficult for you to stay in a room with fluorescent or bright lights? Do you perceive light in an intense way? When did you start to perceive light in this way?

....

....

....

....

....

6. Are you acutely aware of specific sounds and the volume of some sounds? Is it difficult for you to stay in a noisy environment? When did this difficulty start?

....

....

....

....

....

7. Do you like listening to music? Do you like the music to be very loud? Which aspect do you like most in your preferred music?

....

....

....

....

....

8. Do you have difficulty perceiving the internal sensations in your body?

....

....

....

. . . .

. . . .

9. Do you have difficulty with manual activities and motor coordination? When did this difficulty start?

. . . .

. . . .

. . . .

. . . .

. . . .

10. Do you have difficulty perceiving spatial distances and/or distinguishing right from left?

. . . .

. . . .

. . . .

. . . .

. . . .

11. Do you experience your emotions in an intense way?

. . . .

. . . .

. . . .

. . . .

. . . .

H. Health

1. Do you have or have you ever had sleep problems?

. . . .

. . . .

✳

. . . .
. . . .
. . . .

2. Do you have or have you ever had gastrointestinal problems?

. . . .
. . . .
. . . .
. . . .
. . . .

3. Did you or do you make use of drugs?

. . . .
. . . .
. . . .
. . . .
. . . .

4. Did you or do you suffer from hormonal problems and/or auto-immune conditions?

. . . .
. . . .
. . . .
. . . .
. . . .

I. Sexuality

1. Delay in exploratory sexual behaviours

. . . .
. . . .

. . . .

. . . .

. . . .

2. Questioning sexual orientation

. . . .

. . . .

. . . .

. . . .

. . . .

3. History of sexual abuse

. . . .

. . . .

. . . .

. . . .

. . . .

4. Boundary issues/limits regarding sexual experiences

. . . .

. . . .

. . . .

. . . .

. . . .

5. Sexual promiscuity or being asexual

. . . .

. . . .

. . . .

*

. . . .

. . . .

6. Gender flexibility, neutrality or conflict

. . . .

. . . .

. . . .

. . . .

. . . .

Index